P9-BVG-862

Aging and Posttraumatic Stress Disorder

Aging and Posttraumatic Stress Disorder

Edited by

Paul E. Ruskin, M.D., and
John A. Talbott, M.D.

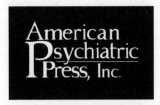

American Psychiatric Press, Inc.

Washington, DC
London, England

Copyright © 1996 American Psychiatric Press, Inc.
ALL RIGHTS RESERVED
Manufactured in the United States of America on acid-free paper
99 98 97 96   4 3 2 1
First Edition

American Psychiatric Press, Inc.
1400 K Street, N.W., Washington, DC   20005

Library of Congress Cataloging-in-Publication Data
Aging and posttraumatic stress disorder / edited by Paul E. Ruskin and
   John A. Talbott. — 1st ed.
      p. cm.
   Includes bibliographical references and index.
   ISBN 0-88048-513-2
   1. Post-traumatic stress disorder in old age.   2. Stress in old
age.   I. Ruskin, Paul E., 1952– .   II. Talbott, John A.
   [DNLM: 1. Stress Disorders, Post-Traumatic—psychology.   2. Aging—
physiology.   3. Veterans—psychology.   4. Models, Biological.
5. Disease Models, Animal.   WM 170 A267 1996]
RC552.P67A36   1996
618.97'68521—dc20
DNLM/DLC
for Library of Congress   95-24078
                                                                                              CIP

British Library Cataloguing in Publication Data
A CIP record is available from the British Library.

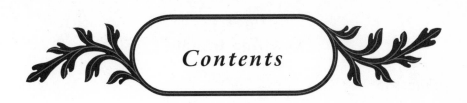

Contents

Part I
Early-Age Trauma and Its Impact on Later Life

Part II
Late-Age Trauma

Part III
Models of Stress in the Elderly

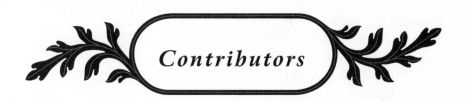

Contributors

Petra G. H. Aarts, M.A.
Psychological Researcher, National Institute for Victims of War (ICODO), Utrecht, Netherlands

Norman B. Anderson, Ph.D.
Associate Professor, Department of Psychiatry, Duke University Medical Center, and Geriatric Research, Education, and Clinical Center, Durham VA Medical Center, Durham, North Carolina

Elizabeth Colerick Clipp, Ph.D., R.N.
Research Assistant Professor of Medicine, Clinical Assistant Professor of Nursing, VA and Duke University Medical Centers, Durham, North Carolina

Johan H. M. De Groen, M.D., Ph.D.
Neurophysiologist, Department of Clinical Neurophysiology, University of Limburg, Maastrict, Netherlands

Glen H. Elder, Jr., Ph.D.
Howard Odum Distinguished Professor of Sociology, Research Professor of Psychology, University of North Carolina at Chapel Hill, Chapel Hill, North Carolina

Paul R. J. Falger, Ph.D.
Psychologist, Department of Medical Psychology, University of Limburg, Maastrich, Netherlands

Robert B. Fields, Ph.D.
Coordinator, Geriatric Psychiatry Program, Allegheny
General Hospital, and Assistant Professor of Psychiatry
(Psychology), Medical College of Pennsylvania and
Hahnemann University, Allegheny Campus, Pittsburgh,
Pennsylvania

Goldine C. Gleser, Ph.D.
Professor Emeritus, Department of Psychiatry, University of
Cincinnati, Cincinnati, Ohio

Marion Zucker Goldstein, M.D.
Clinical Associate Professor, Departments of Psychiatry and
Internal Medicine, State University of New York at Buffalo,
Buffalo, New York

Mary C. Grace, M.Ed., M.S.
Senior Research Associate, Department of Psychiatry,
University of Cincinnati, Cincinnati, Ohio

Bonnie L. Green, Ph.D.
Professor, Department of Psychiatry, Georgetown University,
Washington, D.C.

Charles A. Guarnaccia, Ph.D.
Assistant Professor, Department of Psychology, University of
North Texas, Denton, Texas

Johan E. Hovens, M.D., Ph.D.
Psychiatrist, Centre '45, National Center for the Treatment
of WWII Victims, Oegstgeest, Netherlands

Anthony Leonard, B.A.
Former Research Assistant, Department of Psychiatry,
University of Cincinnati, Cincinnati, Ohio

Jacob D. Lindy, M.D.
Volunteer Associate Professor, Department of Psychiatry,
University of Cincinnati, and the Cincinnati Center for
Psychoanalysis, Cincinnati, Ohio

Maya McNeilly, Ph.D.
Assistant Medical Research Professor, Department of
Psychiatry, Duke University Medical Center, and Center for
the Study of Aging and Human Development, Durham,
North Carolina

Wybrand Op den Velde, M.D., Ph.D.
Psychiatrist, Department of Psychiatry, St. Lucas Hospital,
Amsterdam, Netherlands

Mark J. Rosenthal, M.D.
Staff Physician and Researcher, Geriatric Research,
Education, Clinical Center, Sepulveda Veterans
Administration Medical Center, and Associate Professor,
Department of Medicine, University of California at Los
Angeles, Los Angeles, California

Paul E. Ruskin, M.D.
Associate Professor of Psychiatry, Department of Psychiatry,
University of Maryland, Baltimore, and Chief of Geriatric
Psychiatry, Baltimore VA Hospital, Baltimore, Maryland

John A. Talbott, M.D.
Professor and Chairman, University of Maryland,
Department of Psychiatry, Baltimore, Maryland

Hans Van Duijn, M.D., Ph.D.
Neurophysiologist, Department of Clinical Neurophysiology,
St. Lucas Hospital, Amsterdam, Netherlands

Alex J. Zautra, Ph.D.
Professor, Department of Psychology, Arizona State
University, Tempe, Arizona

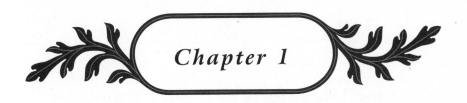

Chapter 1

Introduction

Paul E. Ruskin, M.D., and
John A. Talbott, M.D.

Exposure to natural and human-made disasters can occur at any age in the life cycle. The psychological effects of that exposure, however, may differ depending on the age of the victim at the time of the disaster. Furthermore, the long-term effects of the earlier trauma may change as a person progresses through subsequent developmental stages and into old age. The purpose of this book is to explore both the psychological sequelae of severe trauma in the elderly and the manifestations in old age of psychological symptoms secondary to trauma experienced earlier in life.

Studies of posttraumatic stress disorder (PTSD) are inevitably naturalistic and usually retrospective. A disaster occurs, and investigators try to understand the psychological sequelae. Retrospective, naturalistic studies of this sort are fraught with difficulties. Obtaining data about premorbid level of psychological functioning, determining the amount of stress actually experienced, and identifying a valid control group are difficult tasks to achieve. Nevertheless, several well-designed studies have begun to identify some of the key features of aging and PTSD.

Late-Life Effects of Earlier Trauma

During World War II, millions of people were subjected to overwhelming stress. Soldiers, resistance fighters, prisoners of war, concentration camp victims, and in many localities even the civilian population experienced the daily threat of death, physical injury, and deprivation—often for months or years at a time. This huge cohort of individuals is now entering the later stages of life and offers a priceless opportunity to study late-life psychological effects of earlier trauma.

Assessing the current psychological effects of trauma that occurred 40–50 years ago is, however, a difficult process. A multitude of confounding variables obscures the connection between trauma and symptom. An accurate understanding of the effects of trauma in an individual during World War II would ideally require a great deal of information that is difficult or impossible to obtain. It would be important to know the premorbid level of psychological functioning of the person prior to the onset of the trauma. Were there psychological problems that predated the war? The exact nature, as well as the extent, of the trauma would also be crucial. For instance, was a soldier actively engaged in combat during numerous campaigns or was the soldier stationed in the rear with the supply section? Was the person a passive victim, as were many concentration camp survivors and prisoners of war, or did the person actively participate as a soldier in the killing and maiming? Was the period of stress brief or extended over months and years? Finally, it would be important to know the pattern of symptoms over time. Did the person experience symptoms during the period of stress, shortly after the stress, or only years later? What was the nature of the symptoms and did they change over time?

Is there a subgroup of patients who develop a recurrence of

PTSD symptoms late in life? If so, do psychosocial stresses such as illness, death of a loved one, or retirement from work precipitate the recurrence of symptoms? Finally, what was the nature of the psychosocial supports the patient experienced during the period of stress, just after the period of stress, and in subsequent years?

There are a variety of ways to measure the effects of trauma, particularly trauma that occurred many years before. It is possible, for instance, to investigate current and lifetime rates of PTSD. At the same time, it might also be important to study rates of more general symptoms of psychopathology such as levels of anxiety or depression, social functioning (employment, marriage), and more physiological measures such as sleep disorders. Furthermore, it is important to consider the possibility that a traumatic experience can have positive effects, perhaps by increasing self-confidence or pride of survival.

For obvious reasons, there are no prospective studies that account for all of these confounding variables. Nevertheless, a number of well-designed studies have been conducted with various subgroups of the World War II population. These studies effectively address some, although not all, of the questions about the late-life sequelae of early trauma.

In Chapter 2, Ruskin and Talbott explore the components of successful physiologic and psychologic aging. This chapter serves as a background to subsequent chapters that attempt to answer the question: To what extent can victims of severe trauma age successfully?

In Chapter 3, Clipp and Elder summarize the research that has been conducted with elderly World War II combat veterans. They then present their own work, which is unique in a number of ways. First, their studies benefit from the availability of prewar data of psychological functioning and of a series of assessment points during the course of the years. Also, they view a wide range of outcomes, positive as well as negative. Finally, they investigate the question of whether age at the time of combat affects subsequent outcome.

In Chapter 4, Aarts et al. summarize work that has been done concerning survivors of Nazi persecution during World War II. They then describe their studies of aging Dutch resistance fighters. This work is particularly important because, unlike most studies, these investigators measured PTSD using strict DSM-III-R (American Psychiatric Association 1987) criteria. Also, they present important data on sleep disorders in relationship to late-life PTSD.

Effects of Late-Life Trauma

There are biological, psychological, and social reasons that the elderly might experience psychic trauma differently than younger patients. A number of questions arise concerning possible differences:

- What is the biology of acute and chronic stress in older individuals compared with younger individuals?
- Are there neurophysiologic, hormonal, immunologic, sleep, or other changes observed with severe stress in the elderly that are not observed in younger individuals?
- What is the effect of poor physical health on the manifestation of PTSD symptoms?
- How do developmental issues of late life affect the occurrence and nature of PTSD symptoms?
- How do previous life experiences predispose to, or protect against, the development of PTSD in elderly individuals who are exposed to severe stress?
- What is the treatment for PTSD in the elderly? Does it differ from the treatment for younger patients?

Several studies address some, but not all, of these questions. Cross-sectional studies have compared rates and manifestations of PTSD in the young and elderly exposed to the same natural disaster. A few of these studies even have premorbid information collected retrospectively and a control group of elderly individuals who were not exposed to the disaster.

In Chapter 5, Fields summarizes the literature on PTSD among elderly people exposed to trauma. He suggests that translocation syndrome may be a form of PTSD.

In Chapter 6, Green et al. describe their findings from the well-known Buffalo Creek flood, comparing rates of psychological distress and PTSD among the older segments of the sample to rates in the younger victims. A unique aspect of this study is that there are longitudinal data available at various points in time during a 14-year period.

In Chapter 7, Goldstein examines elder abuse as a possible cause of PTSD. She documents the epidemiology of elder abuse, pointing out how widespread the problem is and profiling the abused and the abuser. She then suggests ways to modify the concept of PTSD to take into account symptoms commonly seen in the elderly.

Models of Stress in the Elderly

Whereas studies of PTSD are of necessity naturalistic, there are three models of stress that have been conducted under more controlled conditions. These provide insight into the relationship between stress and aging, and look at emotional response to life events, physiological response to mild stress, and behavioral and hormonal response to stress in aging animals.

Life Events

There is an extensive literature that examines the effects of life events, chronic stressors, and daily hassles on the psychological well-being of the elderly (George 1989). That literature has become increasingly sophisticated as investigators have realized that there are important factors that mitigate the direct effects of stress on psychological functioning. In particular, strong social support and effective individual coping mechanisms can decrease the impact of a negative life event.

Although the elderly experience fewer stressful life events than younger adults overall, certain events—such as conjugal bereavement, the onset or exacerbation of physical illness, or institutionalization—are more common among the elderly.

In Chapter 8, Guarnaccia and Zautra present results from the Life Events and Aging Project. This longitudinal study of community-dwelling elderly compared psychological sequelae following two common negative life events: the death of a spouse and the onset of a functional disability due to serious illness or injury. Psychological effects are measured sequentially over time in an effort to determine patterns of reactions to these major stressors. Also included in the chapter is an analysis of social supports, coping mechanisms, and the impact of major stressors on the occurrence of positive and negative minor events.

Physiological Measurements

There are numerous physiological differences between the elderly and the young. These differences seem to be more marked in certain organ systems compared with others. Although it would be difficult to study whether the elderly have an increased or decreased physiological response to severe emotional stress such as occurs in PTSD, careful studies have been conducted of mild, laboratory-induced stressors.

In Chapter 9, McNeilly et al. provide an overview of selected, representative studies of age differences in physiological responses to stress. They describe differences in heart rate, blood pressure, electrodermal activity, catecholamine response, and the autonomic nervous system.

Animal Models

Animals models provide a useful means of studying neurophysiologic and hormonal responses to stressful situations.

A number of different mechanisms have been postulated.

In Chapter 10, Rosenthal presents an animal model, describing behavioral and endocrinologic differences in old compared with young rodents exposed to stress. He investigates the role of central and peripheral catecholamines and the hypothalamic-anterior pituitary-adrenal axis. He presents a hypothesis as to how age leads to less active stress response. Finally, he demonstrates how aging might be viewed as a "chronic inescapable stress comparable with that from which a posttraumatic stress disorder originates" (p. 225).

What Can Be Learned About the Nature of Aging and Old Age From a Study of PTSD?

A study of PTSD allows a further examination of the nature of aging and of old age. Two disparate pictures of the elderly exist. One contends that the elderly are frail and vulnerable. This image would suggest that the elderly are more vulnerable to developing PTSD following trauma, that late-life stressors often result in the recurrence of PTSD, that the elderly are more vulnerable to ordinary life stressors than the young, and that the elderly's physiological and endocrinologic response to stress is either inadequate in extent or in modulation.

A different conceptualization of the elderly contends that they are wise and experienced. This image would suggest that the elderly are relatively protected from the effects of severe emotional trauma by a lifetime of dealing with difficult situations. It would postulate that by and large, older people have come to terms with past severe traumas and that only a minority are unable to make their peace with the past. Finally, it would suggest that the elderly's physiological and endocrinologic response to stress is either the same as the young, or perhaps superior because of a diminished response that would result in less symptoms—that is, that the elderly are "calmer," emotionally and physiologically, and therefore less prone to the emotional and physiological displacements that occur with exposure to stress. In this book, we hope to provide an enhanced vision of the elderly and the aging process as applied to stress response.

References

American Psychiatric Association: Diagnostic and Statistical Manual of Mental Disorders, 3rd Edition, Revised. Washington, DC, American Psychiatric Association, 1987

George LK: Stress, social support, and depression over the life-course, in Aging, Stress, and Health. Edited by Markides KS, Cooper CL. New York, Wiley, 1989, pp 241–261

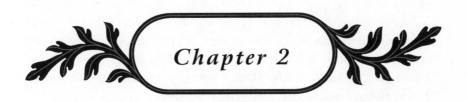

Chapter 2

The Physiology and Psychology of Successful Aging

Paul E. Ruskin, M.D.

T he human organism undergoes dramatic physiological changes during the long journey from birth to old age. Aging—the inexorable process of growing older—begins even before birth, at the moment of conception, and concludes only with the last and final breath.

Physiology

It is obvious that many of the physiological changes that accompany growing older are genetically programmed and therefore innate to the human species. Yet geriatricians continue to be intrigued by a fundamental question: To what extent are the frailties of old age intrinsic to the aging process? And conversely, to what extent are these frailties caused by disease or other external factors—some of which could potentially be controlled and modified?

Many physiological measures show a marked decline with aging. Kidney function, for instance, decreases substantially. Renal blood flow falls by 10% per decade after age 20, and creatinine clearance falls 30% from age 30 to 80 (Tockman 1994). Benign prostatic hypertrophy rarely occurs before age 40, but affects almost 90% of men over the age of 80 (Brendler 1994). Lung function also decreases greatly over time. Forced expiratory volume at one second, for instance, declines 14–30 ml/year in men and 23–32 ml/year in women (Beck 1994).

Physical functioning also declines with age. The ability independently to perform activities of daily living (e.g., bathing, feeding, and toileting) or instrumental activities of daily living (e.g., shopping, using the telephone, and managing money) decreases with age. Whereas at age 65+, 19% of the population has difficulty walking, at age 85, 40% have difficulty. Furthermore, 10% of 65+-year-olds have difficulty with bathing, compared with 28% of 85+-year-olds. Likewise, at age 65+, 7% of the population has difficulty preparing meals, compared with 26% at age 85. Of people age 65+, 5% have difficulty managing money, compared with 24% of those age 85+ (Malmgren 1994). Thus physical—as well as physiological—function declines steadily during the later part of life.

The prevalence of many disabling physical illnesses rises geometrically with age (Mittlemark 1994). For instance, the prevalence of ischemic heart disease increases from 0.2% in men under 45 to 20% in men over 75, and from 0.14% in women under age 45 to 37% in women over age 75. Likewise, the rate of cerebrovascular disease increases from 0.1% in men under age 45 to 7.7% in men over age 75, and from 0.1% in women under age 45 to 6.6% in women over age 75. Perception also declines with age. The rate of visual impairment is 3% for men under age 45 compared with 13% for men over age 75, and 1% for women under age 45 compared with 10% in women over age 75. Hearing impairment occurs in only 4% of men under age 45, compared with 44% over age 75, and in only 3% of women under age 45 compared with 38% in those over age 75.

Thus, as a group, the elderly show a marked decrease in physiological and physical function and a marked increase in the rate of disabling physical illness. Yet one should not assume that all of the elderly are rapidly declining and deteriorating. Indeed, there is much more heterogeneity of function among the elderly than among younger segments of the population. Whereas some elderly are disease ridden and functionally impaired, others are only moderately impaired. There is even a select subgroup that is healthy, able to perform all physical functions well, and physiologically similar to the young (Rowe and Kahn 1987).

External factors unrelated to the aging process per se account for at least some of the observed decline in function and increase in disease among the elderly. For instance, the older person who has smoked cigarettes for 60 years will have poorer lung function and a greater chance of having lung cancer than a comparable older person who has never smoked. Likewise, the liver function of an elderly alcoholic person will probably be worse than that of an elderly nonalcoholic person.

Yet some of the decline seems to be integral to the aging process itself. For instance, even in master athletes who exercise extensively at a high level, there is a gradual decline over the years in maximum heart rate and fat-free weight, as well as an increase in percentage of body weight that is fat (Pollock et al. 1987).

Alzheimer's disease is a paradigmatic example of a geriatric disorder. It is virtually unknown until age 50. Then the prevalence increases exponentially to 45% at age 95 (Miller et al. 1994). It appears to be mainly a genetically programmed disease that does not manifest itself until later in life, much as some of the neurologic disorders of inborn metabolism become apparent at a very early age.

Osteoporosis, a disease process that is very common in elderly women, probably results from a combination of normal aging and external factors. It is associated with menopause, but also with cigarette smoking, poor diet, and lack of exercise. Furthermore, studies indicate that the severity of the disorder can be ameliorated through a combination of proper diet, exercise, and hormonal supplementation or other pharmacological intervention (Krane and Halick 1994).

Who are the successful 85-year-olds, the ones who are free from disabling disease, functionally independent, and physiologically and cognitively fit? A combination of genetic composition (e.g., no genetic predisposition for Alzheimer's disease) and a healthy lifestyle (e.g., lifelong avoidance of smoking, poor diet, excessive alcohol, or a sedentary existence), along with the good fortune to avoid the ravages of major illness or injury, produces successful aging for a lucky minority. One of the major goals of geriatrics is to determine the secret of these successful elderly and to develop interventions that will increase the percentage of future elderly cohorts who fit into this select group.

Psychology

The mind, like the body, is subjected to numerous stresses during the course of a lifetime. There are disappointments and losses. Spouses, friends, and children die. Medical illness, so common in the elderly, limits function and productivity. Social isolation and widowhood, also very common, lead to loneliness and feelings of uselessness. For all of these reasons, it would seem logical that the rate of depression, anxiety, and other psychiatric symptoms would be higher among the elderly than among the young.

Yet research indicates that the rate of psychiatric illness is actually *less* among the elderly. The Epidemiologic Catchment Area (ECA) study, for example, found that the rate of all psychiatric illness in community-dwelling people over the age of 65 was 12.3% compared with 15.4% for the total sample above age 18 (Regier et al. 1988).

Cross-sectional studies indicate that the prevalence of depressive disorders (Regier et al. 1988) and depressive symptoms (Constock and Helsing 1976; Eaton and Kessler 1981;

Frerichs et al. 1981) is lower in elderly than in younger community-dwelling individuals (Blazer 1994). The ECA study
found that whereas the 1-month prevalence of major depression was 2.2% for those above age 18, the rate was only 0.7%
for those above age 65. Likewise, the rate of dysthymia was
1.8% for the elderly compared with 3.3% for those over age
18 years.

The prevalence of anxiety disorders also shows a slight decline with age. The ECA study found that the 1-month prevalence for all anxiety disorders was 7.3% for those over age 18
compared with 6.6% for those over age 64. Of the three specific anxiety disorders studied, phobia and panic disorder had
similar prevalences among the young and old, whereas obsessive-compulsive disorder showed slightly lower rates among
the elderly.

Thus, it would seem that psychological distress, as measured by symptoms of depression and anxiety, decreases, or at
least does not increase dramatically with age as do physical
illness and impairment. Despite the aging process and a lifetime of stressors—including the stressors of old age, social isolation, and medical illness—depression and anxiety are no
more common in the elderly than in younger people. Psychological aging thus differs from physiological aging. Apparently
the human spirit is more resilient than the human body.

Many cultures attribute wisdom to old age. Perhaps it is
this accumulated wisdom that allows the elderly to adjust to
life's vicissitudes without becoming overly depressed or anxious. Some may have successfully reached Erikson's (1963)
eighth stage of psychological development: ego integrity. Erikson defined this concept as

> a post-narcissistic love of the human ego—not of the self—
> as an experience which conveys some world order and
> spiritual sense, no matter how dearly paid for. It is the
> acceptance of one's one and only life cycle as something
> that had to be and that, by necessity, permitted of no sub-
> stitutions. (p. 268)

Successful survivors of severe trauma seem to epitomize this acceptance of life as it was, no matter how terrible or stressful. The archives at Yad Vashem in Jerusalem and the Holocaust Memorial in Washington, DC, are filled with the testimonials of Holocaust survivors who have managed to overcome the terrors of the Holocaust and to lead active, productive lives into their later years. From these people, we have much to learn about how to overcome the worst that life can present.

References

Beck LH: Aging changes in renal function, in Principles of Geriatric Medicine and Gerontology, 3rd Edition. Edited by Hazzard WR, Bierman EL, Blass JP, et al. New York, McGraw-Hill, 1994, pp 615–624

Blazer DG: Is depression more frequent in late life? an honest look at the evidence. American Journal of Geriatric Psychiatry 2:193–199, 1994

Brendler CB: Disorders of the prostate, in Principles of Geriatric Medicine and Gerontology, 3rd Edition. Edited by Hazzard WR, Bierman EL, Blass JP, et al. New York, McGraw-Hill, 1994, pp 657–664

Constock GW, Helsing KJ: Symptoms of depression in two communities. Psychol Med 6:551–563, 1976

Eaton WW, Kessler LG: Rates of symptoms of depression in a national sample. Am J Epidemiol 114:528–538, 1981

Erikson EH: Childhood and Society, 2nd Edition. New York, WW Norton, 1963

Frerichs RR, Aneshensel CS, Clark VA: Prevalence of depression in Los Angeles county. Am J Epidemiol 113:691–699, 1981

Krane SM, Halick MF: Metabolic bone disease, in Harrison's Principles of Internal Medicine, 13th Edition. Edited by Isselbacher KJ, Braunwald E, Wilson JD, et al. New York, McGraw-Hill, 1994, pp 2172–2183

Malmgren R: Epidemiology of aging, in The American Psychiatric Press Textbook of Geriatric Neuropsychiatry. Edited by Coffey CE, Cummings JL. Washington, DC, American Psychiatric Press, 1994, pp 17–33

Miller BL, Chang L, Oropilla G, et al: Alzheimer's disease and frontal lobe dementia, in The American Psychiatric Press Textbook of Geriatric Neuropsychiatry. Edited by Coffey CE, Cummings JL. Washington, DC, American Psychiatric Press, 1994, pp 389–404

Mittlemark MB: The epidemiology of aging, in Principles of Geriatric Medicine and Gerontology, 3rd Edition. Edited by Hazzard WR, Bierman EL, Blass JP, et al. New York, McGraw-Hill, 1994, 135–151

Pollock ML, Foster C, Knap D, et al: Effect of age and training on aerobic capacity and body composition of master athletes. J Appl Physiol 62:725–731, 1987

Regier DA, Boyd JH, Burke JD, et al: One-month prevalence of mental disorders in the United States. Arch Gen Psychiatry 45:977–986, 1988

Rowe JW, Kahn RL: Human aging: usual and successful. Science 237:143–149, 1987

Tockman MS: Aging of the respiratory system, in Principles of Geriatric Medicine and Gerontology, 3rd Edition. Edited by Hazzard WR, Bierman EL, Blass JP, et al. New York, McGraw-Hill, 1994, pp 555–564

Part I

Early-Age Trauma and Its Impact on Later Life

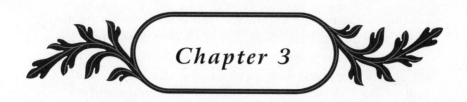

Chapter 3

The Aging Veteran of World War II

Psychiatric and Life Course Insights

Elizabeth Colerick Clipp, Ph.D., R.N., and
Glen H. Elder, Jr., Ph.D.

"Some recollections never die. They lie in one's subconscious, squirreled away, biding their time."

—*Marine Veteran of Okinawa, World War II*
(Manchester 1980, p. 21)

Four decades have passed since the onset of World War II. Most combat soldiers endured fear of death. Large numbers were wounded, witnessed the death of comrades, or lived through periods of captivity. For the majority of young men who survived such experiences, homecoming entailed major adjustments with attempts to reassemble former lives in terms of work, marriage, and family

This chapter is based on a program of research on military service in aging and health. We acknowledge with gratitude financial support from the Veterans Affairs Merit Review Program (E. C. Clipp and G. H. Elder Jr., Co-PIs), from Grant MH 41327 on military service in adult development and aging (G. H. Elder Jr., PI), and from a Research Scientist Award to G. H. Elder Jr.

life. Some veterans made relatively smooth transitions to civilian life, whereas others struggled with emotional problems of various proportion. As the years passed, these men moved through midlife, raised children, and retired from work. Currently, a massive wave of veterans numbering nearly 11 million, approximately half the United States males over the age of 60, are entering their later years. How are these older veterans functioning in the 1990s when compared with nonveterans? To what extent have the emotional wounds of combat healed, become chronic sources of discomfort, or perhaps reopened after years of symptom-free living?

We approach these questions by bringing together evidence from psychiatric research on combat-related symptoms and from life course studies. A life course perspective moves beyond characteristics of the veteran and combat-related symptoms to the broader consequences of war in veterans' lives. Our work in this area is longitudinal and builds on detailed life histories that span many years. Subjects were initially interviewed in adolescence. Subsequent interviews were conducted at a variety of points in the life span (Elder 1974, 1985, 1991). We linked military experience in World War II, especially combat, to life prospects, social ties, and patterns of aging (Elder and Clipp 1988a, 1988b, 1989). In contrast to a psychiatric perspective, which begins with pathology in the individual and then traces backward to etiology, a life course approach begins with an event such as war and traces forward the proximal and distal effects of that event or social change in lives. By examining evidence from both perspectives, clinical and life course, we seek a more detailed portrait of the aging World War II veteran.

Early Studies of Combat-Related Symptoms

The "shell shock" cases observed during and after World War I initiated research in psychological malfunctioning as a result of combat (for reviews, see Brown 1976). Interest in this problem waned between World War I and World War II, as if symptoms subsided with the end of hostilities. An exception to this lack of interest was Kardiner's (1941) work on chronic cases of war neurosis among World War I veterans. He noted a set of "common symptoms," observable in all cases of traumatic neurosis. Symptoms included irritability and startle pattern, fixation on the trauma, atypical dream life, tendency toward explosive and aggressive reactions, and contraction of ego functioning. This pioneering work anticipated a new wave of studies initiated during and after World War II.

Slater (1943) described a "neurotic constitution" as a predisposing risk factor among military personnel, and Symonds (1943) argued that the most important element of "flying stress" in neurosis was exposure to danger. Both analysts concluded that if a family psychiatric history or hereditary factors were present in a particular recruit, neurotic breakdown could be expected under mild combat stress, whereas in the absence of positive family heredity, severe stress was needed to produce symptoms of this kind.

Combat Stress During World War II and in the Postwar Period

What constituted a neurotic breakdown among World War II military? Perhaps the most vivid clinical description of men who became victims is offered by Swank (1949), who studied more than 4,000 cases of combat exhaustion:

> The initial complaint of almost all the men who developed combat exhaustion was persistent fatigue. This was soon followed by the common symptoms of anxiety, namely, a feeling of inadequacy with respect to all tasks, a feeling of insecurity, a tendency to seclusiveness and a fear of crowds. They avoided anything new or different and many feared the prospect of leaving or losing their buddy. All patients exhibited emotional tension. They were easily ir-

ritated and responded quickly. Emotional displays of cry-
ing, laughing, pugnaciousness or moodiness were common, appearing to act as a safety valve for the patient's
tension. (p. 482)

Some kept busy and others drank to excess. They fell
asleep with difficulty, often staying up until very late in
the hope that extreme fatigue might help them in this matter. Dreams were an almost common complaint. Almost all
of the men jumped suddenly when unexpected noises occurred. Retardation was manifested by the slow responses
to questioning and apparent dullness. Memory deficits
were present to the extent that men could not be counted
on to carry out simple orders. (p. 483)

The soldier appeared and acted as if he had lost all feeling.
Somatic symptoms were secondary to anxiety with head
pain the most frequent complaint. Giddiness was frequently associated with headache, described as a feeling of
unsteadiness, uncertainty, or even unreality. Gastric distress was usually associated with anorexia and heart burn,
and in more severe cases with vomiting. Back pain was
common. (p. 486)

Hysterical symptoms consisted of stuttering, aphonia, amnesia and weakness. Muscle tone was depressed, the joints
were flail-like. (p. 488)

Swank (1949) concluded by noting that

we had a willing, healthy young man, probably more stable
than the average civilian, exposed to constant emotional
tension resulting from continual fear of death and uncertainty. To this was added the factor of "blast concussion."
The syndrome which resulted is referred to as combat exhaustion. (p. 505)

Postwar research continued to focus on psychiatric casualties of combat. Weinberg (1946) described "combat neurosis" in terms of confusion, apprehension, impaired attentive ability, irritability, restlessness, apathy, aversion to noise, and nightmares. In addition, however, Weinberg documented postwar social dysfunction connected to the disorder. He noted loss of confidence, self-condemnation, aversion for crowds, an inability to sustain conversation, and intensified cravings for familiar persons and environments and for affection. He described a relationship between neurotic breakdowns during war and a history of childhood problems, but also acknowledged that "a certain proportion of normal and healthy soldiers also succumbed" (p. 465).

Etiological considerations.   Attempting to identify specific psychological predispositions to "operational fatigue" among 284 air crew officers, Grinker et al. (1946a) found that victims of the disorder were significantly more likely than control subjects to report histories of neurotic family background, irritability, minor depressions, feelings of inferiority or homesickness, obsessive and compulsive personality traits, and weaker control of anxiety. Grinker's team of investigators repeated the study using enlisted men and found that enlisted flying personnel with operational fatigue were in many ways comparable to officers with the disorder. However, they noted several differences. The enlisted men more often reported parental discord, broken homes, parental alcoholism, unhappy childhoods, and difficulty with siblings (Grinker et al. 1946b).

Swank (1949) acknowledged the evidence for premilitary personality disturbance among victims of "combat exhaustion," but leaned more toward contextual explanations for the disorder. For example, among more than 2,000 cases of the disorder, he found that problems developed only after severe or prolonged combat. He also found that symptoms could be predicted by the unit casualty rate, suggesting that a fear of death played a critical role in the development of symptoms.

In studies of veterans of both world wars, Kardiner (1941,

1947) suggested that traumatic war neurosis may be the most common psychiatric diagnosis in the world. They referred to the trauma response as "physioneurosis" because symptoms were both psychological and physiological.

Course of Symptoms Over Time: Early Studies

The category of "gross stress reactions" was included in the first DSM (American Psychiatric Association 1952). It was believed that symptoms were transient and reversible. During the 1950s and 1960s, stress research shifted away from issues of diagnosis to questions about the course of the disorder over time.

During the next 25 years, the chronicity of war-related stress symptoms was documented in several important follow-up studies of World War II combat veterans and prisoners of war (POWs). Among 200 psychiatric patients examined in 1950, Futterman and Pumpian-Mindlin (1951) found a 10% prevalence of traumatic war neurosis and a high association between the experience of war atrocities and persistent psychological symptomatology. Surprisingly, many of these men had not, even 5 years after the war, sought treatment for war-related emotional problems. Several years later, Brill and Beebe (1956) found evidence to support a more sophisticated model of "psychoneurosis." Their model included both personal and contextual influences. They observed persistent mental health disturbance among approximately 1,500 World War II veterans who had experienced psychoneurotic breakdown during World War II. Compared with nonpsychiatric control subjects from World War II and the Korean war, victims of the disorder had chronic functional impairment, poorer premilitary adjustment, and more disruptive childhoods. However, they also had more military stressors and exposure to combat.

· In the first follow-up of POWs, Cohen and Cooper (1955) found excess morbidity among prisoners held in Japan. Little or no excess morbidity or mortality was seen in veterans interned in Germany. According to Zeiss and Dickman (1989),

Pacific POWs experienced much more severe treatment and a much longer internment than European POWs. Consistent with this difference, statistics from C. A. Stenger (unpublished data, 1984) cited by Zeiss and Dickman showed that 40% of the men held by the Japanese died in captivity compared with only 1% of the POWs in German camps. Differential outcomes for POWs depending on location of internment are a strong, consistent theme in subsequent work on POWs.

Follow-up studies continued to provide evidence of chronic impairment in many veterans who had been exposed to war stress. Two investigations by Archibald et al. (1962) and Archibald and Tuddenham (1965) lengthened the time frame in which such problems were observed. In the first study, conducted 17 years after World War II, the authors identified a disorder characterized by startle reaction, sleep difficulties, dizziness, blackouts, avoidance of activities similar to combat experience, and internalization of feelings. The second follow-up documented continued and even increased symptomatology 20 years after the war. Moreover, the combat stress group reported more difficulties than control subjects with family and work responsibilities, and about 20% of the symptomatic group reported alcohol problems. Archibald and Tuddenham concluded that the "gross stress syndrome" among veterans is highly persistent over long periods and seems resistant to modification.

In a retrospective study of 303 World War II combat veterans, Hocking (1970) found that more than half of the veterans were significantly disturbed by thoughts of wartime experiences, and many repressed the trauma by somatizing emotional problems.

Physiological Measures of Distress

The 1960s witnessed a rising popularity of laboratory-based behavioral research. Dobbs and Wilson (1960) exposed three groups of men (combat veterans judged socially compensated, combat veterans judged socially decompensated, and noncombatant control subjects) to a tape recording of artillery barrage, small arms fire, and aerial bombardments. In the last half of the recording, single light flashes were added, synchronized with the explosions. Compared with noncombatants, increases in physiological measures (e.g., pulse, respirations, electroencephalographic tracings) occurred in both groups of combat veterans in response to the simulation. Particularly notable were the reactions of members of the socially decompensated group, men whose unsatisfactory work adjustment and psychiatric symptomatology dated from the time of combat. Many of these men could not complete the experiment and left the setting. The inability of some men to complete the experiment was unexpected. The authors concluded that the sounds and sights of combat were conditioned stimuli that induced self-preservation emotional responses of fight, flight, or paralysis. This response was still very strong 15 years after the war. With some modifications, this model has been replicated twice on Vietnam veterans (e.g., Blanchard et al. 1982; Malloy et al. 1983). Findings from these studies support Kardiner's (1941) thesis that symptoms of chronic PTSD result from "conditioning." More recently, Kolb (1984) interpreted the findings as "a conditioned stimulus attachment of overwhelming or long continued fear, inducing combat stimuli to the infantile startle reflex" (p. 241).

Posttraumatic Stress and Vietnam

Research in the 1970s shifted away from veterans of World War II to psychiatric casualties of Vietnam. Indeed, the "Vietnam syndrome" became a major topic of study (Borus 1973, 1974; Egendorf et al. 1981; Helzer et al. 1987; Lifton 1973; Robins et al. 1974), and this interest continues, providing strong consensus that both combat experience and exposure to atrocities hold negative life consequences (DeFazio 1975; Haley 1974; Strange and Brown 1970).

Following the Vietnam War, both researchers and clinicians observed similar human responses to other overwhelming and uncontrollable traumatic situations such as rape, child abuse, and natural disasters. Victims of various ages, with a range of backgrounds and personal resources, appeared to manifest similar responses after experiencing a traumatic event that was "out of the range of usual human experience." Posttraumatic stress disorder (PTSD) was therefore included in DSM-III (American Psychiatric Association 1980) as a separate diagnostic category.

Research on Vietnam veterans gained precision from these formal criteria and continued to dominate the PTSD literature in the early 1980s. However, a number of clinical case studies on older veterans with the disorder also appeared and refocused attention on survivors of World War II.

Delayed PTSD Among World War II Veterans

The term *delayed* PTSD was coined to describe veterans with an apparent first onset of symptoms in later life. A number of examples of delayed response appear in case reports. Christenson et al. (1981) described a 55-year-old veteran who developed symptoms of PTSD after being exposed to a deceased 9-year-old boy in an emergency room where he worked. His history revealed that he had been forced to shoot a 10-year-old boy in the South Pacific because it had been suspected that the Japanese had wired the boy as a human bomb.

Another case, offered by Hamilton (1982), describes a 55-year-old veteran of Okinawa who was admitted for treatment with no memory of having destroyed his apartment and threatened his girlfriend's life. Facts of the case suggest that the stress of deciding whether or not his girlfriend's pregnancy should be terminated reactivated unresolved conflicts stemming from having witnessed the senseless deaths of a woman and child during World War II. Both of these cases illustrate intense survivor guilt, repressed for decades.

Van Dyke et al. (1985) reported the case of a 61-year-old veteran of the European theater. The patient had no precombat psychopathology and enjoyed a long symptom-free interval during which time he pursued a successful architectural career and raised a family. Combat nightmares and periods of depression accompanied deterioration of his health and subsequent retirement. In this stressful context, he became almost totally preoccupied with frightening memories of World War II. The authors concluded that these memories "had been out of his awareness for over 30 years, and that he remembered in exquisite detail and with affects more intense than he had allowed himself on the battlefield" (p. 1072).

Another case of delayed PTSD is presented by Brockway (1988), who described a 66-year-old World War II veteran who participated in 3 months of heavy combat on the border between Germany and Holland. After more than 40 years of healthy functioning, he drank heavily one evening after viewing two war movies. He then experienced a dissociative episode during which he found himself in a dark closet pushing against the door, believing the opposing force on the door was a German soldier. It was his wife.

These and other isolated reports (Kline and Rausch 1985; Pary et al. 1986; Richmond and Beck 1986) provide vivid examples of the intensity of wartime memories and the range of psychological responses to their reactivation. Clinical reports suggest that age-associated losses such as retirement, death of loved ones, children leaving home, or a decline in health can reactivate symptoms of PTSD. Collectively, these declines or losses resemble a prime feature of wartime trauma—a lack of control. It seems that situations in later life that symbolically represent wartime trauma can elicit symptoms that were latent for many years.

Lipton and Schaffer (1986) postulated that age weakens previously adequate defenses. Many of the men adjusted satisfactorily to civilian life, raised families, and were successful in various careers until symptoms intervened. Long lags between stressor and symptoms makes diagnosis of PTSD difficult.

Van der Kolk and Ducey (1984) noted that some retire-ment-age veterans, after years of symptom-free living, experi-ence nightmares about traumatic events in World War II when faced with a loss of structure provided by their jobs. Van der Kolk et al. (1981) surveyed 1,527 veterans ages 25–60+ in a mixed Veterans Administration medical and psychiatric outpa-tient clinic about frequency of nightmares. Of the sample, 30% reported nightmares at least once a month. Combatants ($N =$ 816) had significantly more nightmares than noncombatants ($N = 716$; 38% versus 29%); among the 521 older veterans, 62% reported nightmares at least once a month.

The reasons for the delayed onset of symptoms are unclear, but it has been suggested that some veterans experience a suc-cessful but premature closure on the trauma, which remains dormant until a powerful reminder (Van Dyke et al. 1985) or a breakdown of conscious and unconscious defenses (Kolb 1984) ushers in symptoms. Additional observations by Lipton and Schaffer (1986) on delayed symptoms described how many of these men worked more than one job to induce sleep through exhaustion. In this way they were able to ward off symptoms until increasing age forced a slower pace.

Some authors questioned the existence of delayed PTSD. Shatan (1973) suggested that veterans with apparent delayed PTSD may have been suffering from lingering emotional anes-thesia from combat and that until this emotional anesthesia resolved, PTSD symptoms are hidden. Pary et al. (1986) sug-gested that veterans with apparent delayed PTSD had an on-going subclinical syndrome that became more apparent when the symptoms became more severe.

Recent Studies of War-Related PTSD

The 1980s witnessed a new round of investigations initially aimed at estimating prevalence rates of PTSD for veterans of various wars. Research conducted through the National Viet-nam Veterans Readjustment Study (Kulka et al. 1990) established that the current rate of PTSD among the Vietnam veteran population exposed to combat is approximately 15%, with lifetime rates of about 30%. Results from other studies support these estimates (Card 1983; Egendorf et al. 1981). Unfortunately, the prevalence of PTSD among World War II veterans remains unknown because research to date has not used representative samples.

Helzer et al. (1987) used data from a Midwest site of the Epidemiological Catchment Area Survey (Regier et al. 1984) to examine the prevalence of PTSD among 2,493 participants examined as part of a nationwide general-population survey of psychiatric disorder. The sample included veterans from World War II and the Korean and Vietnam wars. Results suggest that there are 2.4–4.8 million cases of PTSD from all causes in the United States. Helzer et al. suggested that 15% of the males had experienced symptoms of PTSD in their lifetime. However, no combat-related symptoms were reported from veterans of wars other than Vietnam. One possible conclusion from these findings is that PTSD is rare in older veterans. There are, however, other explanations. For one thing, we suspect that men of this era are reluctant to report psychological distress stemming from wartime experiences. Lipton and Schaffer (1986) described the "John Wayne" syndrome in which older veterans are sensitive to not living up to the "ideals of manhood." For men of this generation, psychiatric illness held a negative stigma. They believed that combat neurosis implied psychological weaknesses (Figley 1978) and therefore might be reluctant to report combat-related symptoms. Yet, most will spontaneously cite combat as the most significant stressor in their lives (Rosen et al. 1989).

Another possible explanation is that elderly veterans manifest symptoms of stress somatically rather than psychologically. This potential link between emotional distress and physical symptoms among older veterans receives support in the psychiatric literature (Blake et al. 1990; Butler et al. 1988; Lipton and Schaffer 1986, 1988; Nichols and Czirr 1986). Another possibility is that symptoms of PTSD are misdiagnosed in this population. Nichols and Czirr suggested that PTSD symptoms are frequently misdiagnosed as schizophrenia, alcoholism, antisocial personality disorder, and depression. Clinical interviews by Druley and Pashko (1988) suggest that Korean and World War II veterans with undiagnosed PTSD frequently use alcohol or drugs to control their symptoms and that clinicians have failed to connect the addictive disorders with PTSD. Other veterans with only one or two symptoms of PTSD, such as nightmares (Hendin et al. 1983) or tendency toward aggression (Laufer et al. 1984), may not meet criteria for PTSD diagnosis, yet still are struggling with the legacy of combat. Nichols and Czirr alerted clinicians to the possibility that the symptoms of PTSD might manifest themselves as anxiety or depression because aging clients rarely volunteer details of a traumatic past.

Special Populations

The extent of PTSD among older veterans has been estimated for certain high-risk populations.

Psychiatric and Medical Patients

Rosen et al. (1989) found that 27% of World War II veterans admitted to a geropsychiatric ward suffered from PTSD. Blake et al. (1990) assessed the prevalence of PTSD among 161 nonpsychiatric veteran inpatients on medical units. Of the sample, 70% served in World War II, 13% in the Korean War, and 17% in Vietnam. There were no significant differences in level of combat exposure reported by the three groups. Results showed a 24% overall PTSD rate, with psychiatric disturbance most apparent among Vietnam veterans. Specifically, 46.2% of the Vietnam War group scored in the PTSD range (Mississippi Scale cutoff score of 89) versus 30% of the Korean War group and 18.5% of the World War II veterans.

Former POWs

Several studies have evaluated World War II veterans who were interned by the Germans or Japanese. Distinctive adverse factors of the POW experience (Klonoff et al. 1976) include social isolation, no knowledge or control of destiny, malnutrition, hostile and abusive environment, high incidence of disease with inadequate facilities for treatment, and high death rate. Findings from these studies reveal significant residual psychological and physical sequelae among former POWs. As had been reported by an early study (Cohen and Cooper 1955), veterans imprisoned by the Japanese appeared markedly more symptomatic than those surviving German internment.

Beebe (1975) conducted a medical record follow-up of more than 2,500 POWs of World War II and the Korean War. POWs had significantly higher psychiatric morbidity, psychosocial maladjustment, and physical impairment than era control subjects, and again these differences were significantly more pronounced among men held by the Japanese. POWs interned in Germany showed little evidence of continued ill health.

Zeiss et al. (1985) identified symptom trajectories from clinical surveys administered to World War II and Korean POWs. They found that 20% had symptoms after the war and then again in later life; 36% had symptoms in later life only. They also found that 17% experienced symptoms that faded with time, and 20% were continually affected.

Streimer et al. (1986) noted higher-than-expected rates of suicide among Australian ex-prisoners from the Pacific theater. Dent et al. (1987) compared a random sample of 170 surviving members of the Australian Army who were captured by the Japanese with a random sample of 172 veterans of the same army who fought in Southeast Asia but were not captured. Although there was increased postwar and later-life depression among veterans of both groups who manifested nervous illness during the war, there was a greater postwar prevalence of depressive illness among the POWs and markedly higher depression scale scores 40 years later.

Studies of former World War II POWs reveal high rates of PTSD. Kluznik et al. (1986) performed structured psychiatric examinations on 188 POWs, 153 from Europe and 35 from the Pacific. Lifetime diagnoses of PTSD were made in 67% of these veterans. The presence of PTSD was not correlated with other mental disorders. Similarly, Goldstein et al. (1987) examined 41 former POWs interned by the Japanese. After 40 years, half met full criteria for PTSD, and most reported intrusive memories and nightmares of their time in captivity, as well as interpersonal detachment and difficulties concentrating. Minnesota Multiphasic Personality Inventory data on these men suggest that they have unusual concern for their physical health, a symptom not currently included in the formal PTSD criteria.

Zeiss and Dickman (1989) interviewed a sample of 442 ex-POWs who had been interned by the Germans or Japanese. Overall, 55.7% reported symptoms consistent with a clinical diagnosis of PTSD, with no notable differences by site of internment. The strongest predictor of PTSD symptomatology was rank at the time of capture (men of lower rank experienced more difficulty) rather than severity or duration of captivity. The authors suggested that personal attributes such as greater self-efficacy, intelligence, and maturity may result in rank promotion and ability to cope with stress. With regard to the lack of relationship between location of internment and PTSD, the authors offered two possibilities. First, excessive mortality among Pacific POWs may have attenuated the relationship. Second, PTSD may be a threshold phenomenon such that beyond a certain level, increased duration or severity of trauma does not result in more symptomatology.

A similarly high prevalence rate for PTSD among ex-POWs comes from a study by Speed et al. (1989), who estimated the relative contributions of trauma and premorbid dispositions in the development and persistence of PTSD. Among 62 former POWs of World War II, 50% met criteria for PTSD after repatriation, and 29% continued to meet criteria for the disorder

four decades later. The strongest predictors of PTSD were proportion of body weight lost and the experience of torture in
captivity. These findings thus suggest that familial predisposition and preexisting psychopathology are less important than
the actual trauma of the POW experience. Proportion of weight
loss in captivity has been found by others to predict long-term
compromises in cognitive performance among World War II
POWs (Sutker et al. 1990; Thygesen et al. 1970).

These and other studies of former POWs suggest that long-
term responses to severe and prolonged stress present a complicated interaction of cognitive, behavioral, and emotional
symptoms. For many, the trauma appears to have undermined
aspects of both biological and psychological functioning over
extended periods of time, up to the present. Interestingly, with
the exception of work by Zeiss et al. (1985), delayed onset of
PTSD is not reported among POWs. Symptoms typically
emerged after repatriation and either continued or resolved
over the years. Both personal and contextual characteristics
have been identified as relating to the risk of PTSD among
former POWs, with higher military rank at the time of capture
serving as a protective factor.

Veterans of Pearl Harbor

Harel and Kahana (1989) evaluated 250 survivors of the Japanese attack on Pearl Harbor. Their study population consisted
of members of the Pearl Harbor Survivors Association who at-
tended the 45th reunion of the attack in Hawaii. Of this
group, 65% reported intrusive imagery, 42% described survivor guilt, nearly one-fourth reported startle responses to loud
noises, and one-third still experienced difficulty talking about
the Day of Infamy.

Resistance Fighters

Op den Velde et al. (1990) examined eight survivors of the
Dutch Resistance who met formal criteria for PTSD. In all

subjects, symptoms occurring in later life were more severe than postwar symptoms.

Comparison of World War II and Vietnam Veterans

Among veterans with current PTSD, Davidson et al. (1990) found that those who served in Vietnam were more symptomatic than older veterans of World War II. In addition, their data show a difference by war in what is remembered as stressful or painful. Vietnam veterans recalled brutality, mutilated bodies, death of children, and loss of friends as the worst experiences. In contrast, World War II veterans focused on physical injuries, incapacity, and captivity as the worst experiences. The authors suggested that emotional injury to Vietnam veterans involved interpersonal issues whereas World War II combat veterans perceive their trauma in relation to personal threat.

Treatment

Epstein (1989) provided a thorough review of treatment approaches for veterans with PTSD, including psychodynamic psychotherapy, behavioral therapy, cognitive therapy, group therapy, hypnosis, narcosynthesis, and pharmacotherapy. Choice of a method or combination of approaches depends on the needs of the patient, features of the disorder, presence of external support, and cultural factors. It is currently unclear, however, what the management approach to the aging veteran with PTSD should entail. In an excellent review of PTSD and combat-related symptoms in older veterans, Schnurr (1991) cited this gap in our current knowledge as a major limitation of PTSD research.

Limitations of Cross-Sectional Studies

The literature on PTSD in World War II veterans is limited in a number of ways. Most of the studies are cross-sectional and rely on retrospective reporting of both war experiences and symptom patterns through the years. Most of the data are provided either through case reports or descriptions of nonrandom samples of clinical or other special populations. There are no good community-based samples, and most of the studies did not use control groups. Few data are available on prewar psychological functioning. Finally, the potential effects of combat are narrowly defined and focus only on symptoms of PTSD or other psychiatric symptoms or both. The broader psychosocial consequences of combat experiences are generally not considered.

Life Course Studies of Military Experience and Aging

Longitudinal, life course studies remedy some of the deficits of cross-sectional studies. They allow for assessment of the effects of precombat functioning on the development of postcombat symptoms. They provide more complete assessment of symptom patterns over time. Finally, they allow for a broader consideration of combat-related psychosocial effects across the life span.

Data for our studies of military experience and aging come from three archives with prospective and retrospective life record data: the Oakland Growth Study (birth years, 1920–1921), the Berkeley Guidance Study (birth years, 1928–1929), and the Lewis Terman Study (birth years, 1904–1920). Of the Oakland men, 90% served in the armed forces, compared with 73% of the Berkeley men and 45% of the Terman men. We divided each cohort by combat experience (none, light, or heavy) to trace effects of this experience prospectively into the later years. Multiple follow-ups across the early, middle, and later years have allowed us to examine prewar factors, aspects of military experience, and the short- and long-term effects of war in multiple dimensions.

Premorbid Factors

Using California Q-sort ratings in adolescence for the Oakland and Berkeley men, we found that men who were at greatest risk of stress symptoms in the postservice era ranked higher in adolescence on self-inadequacy, introspectiveness, and a lack of ego resilience, when compared with other men. Moreover, we found that combat veterans who were resilient adolescents tended to show more gains in ego resilience up to midlife than servicemen who ranked low on adolescent resilience (Elder and Clipp 1989). Ego resilience tended to moderate the stressful effects of wartime combat, just as an introspective orientation enhanced the risk of enduring stress reactions.

Three-quarters of the veterans with emotional problems after service experienced nightmares in late childhood. Eight of the men who served in heavy combat had prior records of sleep disturbances. Of this number, four experienced postservice problems (depression, inability to concentrate, intense anxiety, intrusive memories, nightmares), and four had a childhood history of nightmares (as distinguished from night terrors). Three men with no emotional problems after the service showed no evidence of nightmares in late childhood (Elder and Clipp 1988a).

Exposure to combat and social ties. As evidenced repeatedly in cross-sectional, retrospective studies, we found that men who experienced heavy combat during World War II were also veterans with a high risk of emotional and behavioral problems following the war. This risk diminishes over time, but it persists into later life (Elder and Clipp 1988a). Using life-history data from the 1985 follow-up of the Oakland and

Berkeley subjects and spouses, we found degree of combat experience to be highly correlated with reports of stress symptoms, traumatic memories, and guilt over survival (Elder and Clipp 1988a, 1988b). Heavy combat veterans were most likely to report emotional and behavioral problems on leaving the service (over 50%), and those who reported emotional problems at that time were more likely than other men to acknowledge war-linked symptoms in later life (25% versus 7%). This contrast is even greater on the question of whether military and wartime service was ever too painful to think about (55% versus 14%).

In the later years, memories of war trauma were associated with severity of combat experience: the heavier the combat, the more common the intrusive memories (Elder and Clipp 1988a). Men who scored highest on trauma memories were more likely than others to be connected with service buddies and to have spouses who knew and understood their legacy of the war. From the 1940s to the present, a number of men improved (i.e., reported fewer symptoms of PTSD). The men who reported having a supportive community of wartime comrades and a supportive wife who understood her husband's war-related problems tended to improve the most. Ironically, war trauma characterized by loss of friends contributed strongly to the formation of this community, which in turn diminished the war-related symptoms of stress. We have found that reunions of a military unit can be an important part of veteran healing.

Our studies showed that veterans exposed to combat deaths (subgroup of heavy combat veterans) in World War II were more likely than others to report enduring services ties (Elder and Clipp 1988b). Stress symptoms were most common among subjects who experienced *both* combat and the loss of a buddy. The greater the war trauma, as indicated by loss of comrades and by general stress reactions, the stronger the link between the service and enduring social relationships with men from their military units. These ties include the exchange of letters and cards, phone calls, and visits. The veterans with these long-term relationships from the war were most likely to participate in occasional reunions of their primary military group.

Finally, we found severity of combat in World War II to be more strongly predictive of physical rather than emotional problems at later ages (Elder et al. 1993). This pattern of physical impairment and decline resembles an accelerated form of aging.

Benefits

Interestingly, when we examined the meaning of combat in later life, we found that heavy combat veterans have mixed memories of losses and life benefits from military experience, suggesting that the effects of combat may not only impair but also enhance personal growth.

Approximately 15 years after World War II, a former Marine in the Berkeley sample who had four landings in the South Pacific talked about the nightmares that tormented him, the "hollering and screaming in the middle of the night." Ten years later, he observed that "I can close my eyes and feel the water under my arms. . . . the fear was awful. . . . it took every bit of energy I could summon, every bit of self-control, for me to get out of the landing boat. . . . I was so scared I had nightmares for years." However, when asked in his 50s whether the service had made any difference in the kind of person he became, this veteran stressed that through combat he had learned the ability to survive adversity—"all one needs is the will to survive— and the skill to cooperate with others and to be dependable and self-disciplined" (for additional case material, see Elder and Clipp 1988a).

Timing of mobilization. Wartime mobilization typically seeks young men and women in their late teens and early 20s who are not yet involved in families and career. However, human resources pressures during World War II resulted in the recruitment of many older recruits in their late 20s and early 30s. A comparison of early-age and late-age recruits allowed us to determine which group had more psychiatric and psychosocial problems associated with being in combat.

Stouffer (1949a, 1949b) showed that young soldiers in World War II were at a higher risk of stress reactions than their older peers. Work by Hastings (1991) using the Terman men supports this conclusion. He found that older veterans had a lower incidence of emotional problems in 1950 than did younger veterans (7% versus 17%) and that this contrast was similar in 1960 (14% versus 22%). In neither group did the soldiers have evidence of impaired emotional health before the war.

On the other hand, we found numerous socioeconomic disadvantages associated with late-age recruitment. We hypothesize that early entry into the military tended to maximize service benefits by preceding family and career obligations, opening up educational benefits from the GI Bill, and fostering developmental growth. The later the mobilization, the greater the conflict between military obligations and civilian pursuits, especially those of family and career. All empirical findings on time of entry support this hypothesis for the Oakland and Berkeley cohorts (Elder 1986, 1987; Elder and Bailey 1988). Exposure to combat in both cohorts is unrelated to time of entry. Furthermore, men mobilized early in their lives tended to be more disadvantaged on family background than late entrants, especially in relation to Depression hardship. They also ranked lower in adolescence on school performance and self-adequacy than later entrants. However, by middle age, occupational differences between late-age and early-age entrants were largely nonexistent. The early entrants generally matched the occupational standing of the late entrants. Late entrants often encountered problems in restarting their interrupted careers after leaving the service.

Using Q-sort ratings of personality in adolescence and at midlife for the Berkeley men, we found that developmental change toward greater self-direction, confidence, and assertive-

ness characterized the early entrants compared with late entrants and nonveterans. Time of entry provided some basis for
understanding how men from economically hard-pressed families in the 1930s managed to equal the socioeconomic achievements of late-entry men from more privileged, nondeprived
homes. Even the initially adverse effects associated with low-
resource childhoods among the Berkeley males seemed to have
been canceled by the gains (e.g., use of the GI Bill) and developmental changes (e.g., increased maturity and independence)
associated with early entry into the service. Subjects in the
Terman sample were born between 1904 and 1920, and therefore entered World War II at a much later point in the life
course than the Berkeley and Oakland men. As a result, we
expected more pronounced socioeconomic disadvantages
among the late entrants. As in the other two samples, later
entrants among the Terman sample, especially men in professional careers who entered the service after the age of 29,
tended to encounter an enduring economic disadvantage in
terms of lost earnings when compared with nonveterans (Hastings 1988). The economic disadvantage remained across the
middle years, and older veterans never completely made up the
losses from their wartime service. This difference between
older and younger veterans was not due to preservice attributes, such as father's occupational status and their own IQ.
In comparison to younger nonveterans, younger veterans
caught up early and achieved a modest economic advantage
that they maintained throughout their careers. A research
chemist in the older veteran group illustrates the costs of the
draft at age 32. After the war, he described how his military
experience left him behind on technical skills. Ten years later,
he still felt the gaps in his career development and decided to
shift into administration.

In an analysis that focused on the relationship between
military service and marital disruption (Pavalko and Elder
1990), we found that veterans were more likely to divorce than
nonveterans. For veterans who were married by time of entry,
the risk of divorce was greater among those who entered the

service relatively late in life and for those who experienced combat. Specifically, married men who were over the age of 30 when they entered the service were more likely to be divorced by 1955 than younger married recruits. We believe this differential reflects the age-related obligations for men in family and work and thus the more disruptive consequences of war for later-age entrants.

The departure of husbands posed a serious problem for wives and their children in terms of economic support and family life, as did the return of veterans to families that had learned to cope without them. The breakdown of marital relations in the postwar years has important implications for the social and emotional adjustment of veterans to civilian life, for men's work life, and for the family support and integration of men in later life.

Overall, our studies on timing of mobilization suggest that older recruits show more serious long-term career and family consequences from the war because of the crucial point at which their lives were interrupted. Younger soldiers, however, may suffer more psychological consequences of military experience due, perhaps, to less mature coping abilities.

Conclusion

Wartime experiences acquire an element of immortality through their imprint on survivors. There are approximately 11 million American veterans of World War II, all of whom are currently entering the geriatric age group. Several million of these veterans experienced combat, and 1 in 200 servicemen were captured as POWs (Nichols and Czirr 1986).

Evidence from clinical reports, surveys of a number of different types of nonrandomly selected populations (former POWs, resistance fighters, geropsychiatric patients, survivors of Pearl Harbor), and longitudinal studies based on three extensive archives suggest that a portion of elderly combat veterans are at risk for the development or exacerbation of PTSD symptoms, perhaps in part because of the losses and stresses of aging. Various longitudinal patterns of symptom presentation have been identified, including symptoms during or shortly after the war with resolution, ongoing symptoms since the time of the war, and onset of symptoms in late life. Overall, the extent of symptomatology seems to have diminished with time.

Predictors of later-life symptomatology include poorer psychological functioning in adolescence, greater degree and severity of combat exposure, a history of psychological symptoms during the immediate postwar period, and postwar lack of emotional support from wives and former comrades. Former POWs seem to manifest a high rate of PTSD. Life course studies document the increased social disruption to late-entry compared with early-entry veterans.

The large cohort of aging veterans offers an excellent opportunity to understand the impact of severe trauma in early adulthood on adjustment in later life. A number of important research questions remain unanswered. Community-based studies are needed to determine the rate of PTSD in elderly veterans compared with nonveterans and to determine if there is a relationship between late-life stressors and the exacerbation of PTSD.

Treatment-outcome studies are needed to document the best form or forms of treatment for PTSD in elderly veterans. Ongoing longitudinal studies are also important to document the full range of war-related symptomatology and life course effects throughout the course of old age.

Finally, there is evidence that PTSD in World War II veterans is currently underdiagnosed because of an unwillingness on the part of veterans to associate current symptoms with war experiences. Symptomatology is sometimes misdiagnosed as anxiety, alcoholism, depression, or schizophrenia. Clinicians should routinely ask geriatric patients about their military history and should consider the possibility of combat-related PTSD in patients having a history of combat. More accurate assessment could lead to better psychiatric treatment for this large cohort of elderly veterans.

References

American Psychiatric Association: Diagnostic and Statistical Manual: Mental Disorders. Washington, DC, American Psychiatric Press, 1952

American Psychiatric Association: Diagnostic and Statistical Manual of Mental Disorders, 3rd Edition. Washington, DC, American Psychiatric Press, 1980

Archibald HC, Tuddenham RD: Persistent stress reaction after combat: a 20-year follow-up. Arch Gen Psychiatry 12:475–481, 1965

Archibald HC, Long DM, Miller C, et al: Gross stress reaction in combat: a 15-year follow-up. Am J Psychiatry 119:317–322, 1962

Beebe GW: Follow-up studies of World War II and Korean war prisoners, II: morbidity, disability, and maladjustments. Am J Epidemiol 101:400–422, 1975

Blake DD, Keane TM, Wine PR, et al: Prevalence of PTSD symptoms in combat veterans seeking medical treatment. Journal of Traumatic Stress 3:15–27, 1990

Blanchard EB, Kolb LC, Pallmeyer TP, et al: A psychological study of post traumatic stress disorder in Vietnam veterans. Psychiatr Q 54:220–229, 1982

Borus JF: Reentry: II: "making it" back in the States. Am J Psychiatry 130:850–854, 1973

Borus JF: Incidence of maladjustment in Vietnam returnees. Arch Gen Psychiatry 30:554–557, 1974

Brill NQ, Beebe GW: A Follow-Up Study of War Neuroses (VA Medical Monograph). Washington, DC, Veterans Administration, 1956

Brockway S: Case report: flashback as a post-traumatic stress disorder (PTSD) symptom in a World War II veteran. Milit Med 153:372–373, 1988

Brown MW: Neuropsychiatry and the War: A Bibliography With Abstracts. Edited by Williams FE. New York, Arno, 1976

Butler RW, Roy DW, Snodgrass L, et al: Post-traumatic stress disorder in a combat-related nonpsychiatric population. Journal of Anxiety Disorders 2:111–120, 1988

Card JJ (ed): Lives After Vietnam: The Personal Impact of Military Service. Lexington, MA, Lexington Books, 1983

Christenson RM, Walker JI, Ross DR, et al: Reactivation of traumatic conflicts. Am J Psychiatry 138:984–985, 1981

Cohen BM, Cooper MZ: A Follow-Up Study of World War II Prisoners of War (United States Veterans Administration Medical Monograph). Washington, DC, Superintendent of Documents, U.S. Government Printing Office, 1955

Davidson JRT, Kudler HS, Saunders WB, et al: Symptom and comorbidity patterns in World War II and Vietnam veterans with posttraumatic stress disorder. Compr Psychiatry 31: 162–170, 1990

DeFazio VJ: The Vietnam era veteran: psychological problems. Journal of Contemporary Psychotherapy 7:9–15, 1975

Dent OF, Tennant CC, Goulston KJ: Precursors of depression in World War II veterans 40 years after the war. J Nerv Ment Dis 175:486–490, 1987

Dobbs D, Wilson WP: Observations on persistence of war neurosis. Diseases of the Nervous System 21:686–691, 1960

Druley KA, Pashko S: Posttraumatic stress disorder in World War II and Korean combat veterans with alcohol dependency. Recent Dev Alcohol 6:89–101, 1988

Egendorf A, Kadushin C, Laufer RS, et al: Legacies of Vietnam: Comparative Adjustment of Veterans and Their peers—A Study Conducted for the Veterans Administration, Vol 1: Summary of Findings. Washington, DC, U.S. Government Printing Office, 1981

Elder GH Jr: Children of the Great Depression: Social Change in Life Experience. Chicago, IL, University of Chicago, 1974

Elder GH Jr (ed): Life Course Dynamics: Trajectories and Transitions, 1968–1980. Ithaca, New York, Cornell University Press, 1985

Elder GH Jr: Military times and turning points in men's lives. Developmental Psychology 22:233–245, 1986

Elder GH Jr: War mobilization and the life course: a cohort of World War II veterans. Sociological Forum 2:449–472, 1987

Elder GH Jr: The life course, in Encyclopedia of Sociology. Edited by Borgatta EF, Borgatta ML. New York, Macmillan 1991, pp 1120–1130

Elder GH Jr, Bailey S: The timing of military service in men's lives, in Social Stress and Family Development. Edited by Klein DM, Aldous J. New York, Guilford, 1988, pp 157–174

Elder GH Jr, Clipp EC: Combat experience, comradeship, and psychological health, in Human Adaptation to Extreme Stress: From the Holocaust to Vietnam. Edited by Wilson JP, Harel Z, Kahana B. New York, Plenum, 1988a, pp 131–156

Elder GH Jr, Clipp EC: Wartime losses and social bonding: influences across 40 years in men's lives. Psychiatry 51:177–198, 1988b

Elder GH Jr, Clipp EC: Combat experience and emotional health: impairment and resilience in later life. J Pers 57:311–341, 1989

Elder GH Jr, Shanahan JM, Clipp ED: When war comes to men's lives: life course patterns in family, work and health. Psychol Aging 9:5–16, 1993

Epstein RS: Contemporary psychiatry: posttraumatic Stress disorder: a review of diagnostic and treatment issues. Psychiatry Annals 556–563, 1989

Figley CR (ed): Stress Disorders Among Vietnam Veterans: Theory, Research, and Treatment. New York, Brunner/Mazel, 1978

Futterman S, Pumpian-Mindlin E: Traumatic war neuroses five years later. Am J Psychiatry 108:401–408, 1951

Goldstein G, van Kammen W, Shelly C, et al: Survivors of imprisonment in the Pacific theater during World War II. Am J Psychiatry 144:1210–1213, 1987

Grinker RR, Willerman B, Bradley AD, et al: A study of psychological predisposition to the development of operational fatigue, I: in officer flying personnel. Am J Orthopsychiatry 16:191–206, 1946a

Grinker RR, Willerman B, Bradley AD, et al: A study of psychological predisposition to the development of operational fatigue, II: in enlisted flying personnel. Am J Orthopsychiatry 16:207–214, 1946b

Haley SA: When the patient reports atrocities: specific treatment considerations of the Vietnam veteran. Arch Gen Psychiatry 30:191–196, 1974

Hamilton JW: Unusual long-term sequelae of a traumatic war experience. Bull Menninger Clin 46:539–541, 1982

Harel Z, Kahana B: The day of infamy: the legacy of Pearl Harbor, in Trauma, Transformation, and Healing. Edited by Wilson JP. New York, Brunner/Mazel, 1989, pp 129–156

Hastings TJ: The effects of military status on men's career earnings: insights gained from using a life course perspective. Doctoral dissertation, Chapel Hill, NC, University of North Carolina at Chapel Hill, 1988

Hastings TJ: The Stanford-Terman study revisited: postwar emotional health of World War II veterans. Military Psychology 3:201–214, 1991

Helzer JE, Robins LN, McEvoy L: Post-traumatic stress disorder in the general population: findings of the Epidemiologic Catchment Area Survey. N Engl J Med 317:1630–1634, 1987

Hendin H, Haas AP, Singler P, et al: Evaluation of posttraumatic stress in Vietnam veterans. Journal of Psychiatric Treatment and Evaluation 5:303–307, 1983

Hocking F: Psychiatric aspects of extreme environmental stress. Diseases of the Nervous System 31:542–545, 1970

Kardiner A: The traumatic neuroses of war, in Psychosomatic Medicine Monograph II–III. Edited by Hoeber P. Washington, DC, National Research Council, 1941, pp 11–111

Kardiner A: Preface, in War Stress and Neurotic Illness. New York, Hoeber, 1947, pp x–xii

Kline NA, Rausch JL: Olfactory precipitants of flashbacks in posttraumatic stress disorder: case reports. J Clin Psychiatry 46:383–384, 1985

Klonoff H, McDougall GM, Clark C, et al: The neuropsychological, psychiatric, and physical effects of prolonged and severe stress: 30 years later. J Nerv Ment Dis 163:246–252, 1976

Kluznik JC, Speed N, VanValkenburg C, et al: Forty-year follow-up of United States prisoners of war. Am J Psychiatry 143:1443–1446, 1986

Kolb LC: The post-traumatic stress disorders of combat: a subgroup with a conditioned emotional response. Milit Med 149:237–243, 1984

Kulka RA, Schlenger WE, Fairbank JA, et al: Trauma and the Vietnam War Generation: Report of Findings From the National Vietnam Veterans Readjustment Study. New York, Brunner/Mazel, 1990

Laufer RS, Brett E, Gallops MS: Post-traumatic stress disorder (PTSD) reconsidered: PTSD among Vietnam veterans, in Post-Traumatic Stress Disorder: Psychological and Biological Sequelae. Edited by van der Kolk BA. Washington, DC, American Psychiatric Press, 1984, pp 1304–1311

Lifton RJ: Home from the War: Vietnam Veterans—Neither Victims nor Executioners. New York, Simon & Schuster, 1973

Lipton MI, Schaffer WR: Post-traumatic stress disorder in the older veteran. Milit Med 151:522–524, 1986

Lipton MI, Schaffer WR: Physical symptoms related to post-traumatic stress disorder (PTSD) in an aging population. Milit Med 153:316–318, 1988

Malloy PE, Fairbank JA, Keane TM: Validation of a multimethod assessment of posttraumatic stress disorder in Vietnam veterans. J Consult Clin Psychol 51:488–494, 1983

Manchester WR: Goodbye, Darkness:A Memoir of the Pacific War. Boston, Little, Brown, 1980

Nichols BL, Czirr R: Post-traumatic stress disorder: hidden syndrome in elders. Clinical Gerontologist 5:417–433, 1986

Op den Velde W, Falger PRJ, de Groen JHM, et al: Current psychiatric complaints of Dutch resistance veterans from World War II: a feasibility study. Journal of Traumatic Stress 3:351–358, 1990

Pary R, Turns DM, Tobias CR: A case of delayed recognition of posttraumatic stress disorder (letter). Am J Psychiatry 143:941, 1986

Pavalko E, Elder GH: World War II and divorce: a life-course perspective. The American Journal of Sociology 5:1213–1234, 1990

Regier DA, Myers JK, Kramer M, et al: The NIMH Epidemiologic Catchment Area program: historical context, major objectives, and study population characteristics. Arch Gen Psychiatry 41:934–941, 1984

Richmond JS, Beck JC: Posttraumatic stress disorder in a World War II veteran (letter). Am J Psychiatry 143:1485–1486, 1986

Robins LN, Davis DH, Goodwin DW: Drug use by U.S. Army enlisted men in Vietnam: a follow-up on their return home. Am J Epidemiol 99:235–249, 1974

Rosen J, Fields RB, Hand AM, et al: Concurrent posttraumatic stress disorder in psychogeriatric patients. J Geriatr Psychiatry Neurol 2:65–69, 1989

Schnurr PP: PTSD and combat-related psychiatric symptoms in older veterans. PTSD Research Quarterly 2, 1991

Shatan CF: The grief of soldiers: Vietnam combat veterans' self-help movement. Am J Orthopsychiatry 43:640–653, 1973

Slater E: The neurotic constitution. Journal of Neurological Psychiatry 6:1–6, 1943

Speed N, Engdahl B, Schwartz J, et al: Posttraumatic stress disorder as a consequence of the POW experience. J Nerv Ment Dis 177:147–153, 1989

Stouffer SA, Sucman EA, De Vinney LC, et al: The American Soldier, Vol 1: Adjustment During Army Life. Princeton, NJ, Princeton University Press, 1949a

Stouffer SA, Lumsdaine AA, Lumsdaine MH, et al: The American Soldier, Vol 2: Combat and Its Aftermath. Princeton, NJ, Princeton University Press, 1949b

Strange RE, Brown DE: Home from the war: a study of psychiatric problems in Viet Nam returnees. Am J Psychiatry 127:130–134, 1970

Streimer J, Temperly H, Tennant C: The adjustment of hospitalized Vietnam veterans. Aust N Z J Psychiatry 20:77–81, 1986

Sutker PB, Galina ZH, West JA, et al: Trauma-induced weight loss and cognitive deficits among former prisoners of war. J Consult Clin Psychol 58:323–328, 1990

Swank RL: Combat exhaustion. J Nerv Ment Dis 109:475–508, 1949

Symonds CP: The human response to flying stress: Lecture I: neurosis in flying personnel. BMJ 2:703–706, 1943

Thygesen P, Hermann K, Willanger R: Concentration camp survivors in Denmark: persecution, disease, disability, compensation: a 23-year follow-up—a survey of the long-term effects of severe environmental stress. Dan Med Bull 17:65–108, 1970

van der Kolk BA, Ducey C: Clinical implications of the Rorschach in posttraumatic stress disorder, in Posttraumatic Stress Disorder: Psychological and Biological Sequelae. Edited by van der Kolk BA. Washington, DC, American Psychiatric Press, 1984, pp 303–321

van der Kolk BA, Burr WA, Blitz A, et al: Characteristics of nightmares among veterans with combat experience. Sleep Research 10:179–185, 1981

Van Dyke C, Zilberg NJ, McKinnon JA: Posttraumatic stress disorder: a thirty-year delay in a World War II veteran. Am J Psychiatry 142:1070–1073, 1985

Weinberg SK: The combat neuroses. The American Journal of Sociology 51:465–487, 1946

Zeiss RA, Dickman HR: PTSD 40 years later: incidence and person-situation correlates in former POWs. J Clin Psychol 45:80–87, 1989

Zeiss RA, Dickman HR, Nichols BL: Posttraumatic stress disorder in former prisoners of war: incidence and correlates. Paper presented at the 93rd Annual Convention of the American Psychological Association, Los Angeles, CA, August 1985

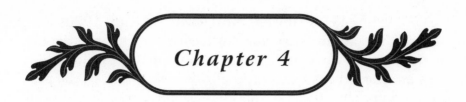

Chapter 4

Late Onset of Posttraumatic Stress Disorder in Aging Resistance Veterans in the Netherlands

Petra G. H. Aarts, M.A.,
Wybrand Op den Velde, M.D., Ph.D.,
Paul R. J. Falger, Ph.D.,
Johan E. Hovens, M.D., Ph.D.,
Johan H. M. De Groen, M.D., Ph.D., and
Hans Van Duijn, M.D., Ph.D.

> "What makes old age hard to bear is not a failing
> of one's faculties, mental or physical, but the bur-
> den of one's memories."
>
> —*Somerset Maugham* (1959, p. 70)

P sychic trauma is a phenomenon that is bound to be as old and common as human-ity itself. It is only since the introduction of posttraumatic stress disorder (PTSD) in DSM-III (American Psychiatric Association 1980), however, that posttraumatic symptomatol-ogy has met with general recognition and acknowledgment. It was the sad condition of those returning from the Southeast

Asian "killing fields" during the 1960s and early 1970s that focused the attention of mental health professionals in the United States on posttraumatic symptomatology. In 1980, this interest led to the conceptualization of PTSD. In the past decennium, the study of the mental and physical effects of psychic trauma expanded remarkably. PTSD, with its core characteristics of alternating intrusive and avoidance symptoms, is now the main focus of interest for research of psychic trauma in the Western world.

Yet, another historical event, not even that far remote from the present days, did not have that effect. After World War II, it only gradually became clear that survivors of Nazi persecution could suffer seriously and persistently as a consequence of what they had been through. Since the first decades after World War II, many clinical and empirical studies—some of them of high quality and sophistication—have been published on survivors of this war. The "survivor syndrome" became a new diagnostic construct, wherein anxiety, depression, insomnia, nightmares, hypermnesia, cognitive disturbances, and somatization were predominant symptoms (Krystal 1968). Not only survivors of labor and concentration camps could suffer from a survivor syndrome, but also military veterans (Kardiner 1941), people who escaped annihilation by hiding or in undercover (Venzlaff 1964), and those who were engaged in activities of resistance against the German occupier (Bastiaans 1957, 1974; Eitinger 1961; Thygesen and Hermann 1954). More recent studies on survivors of Nazi-persecution and World War II military veterans have shown that posttraumatic symptomatology, even more than 40 years after the war, can still be prevalent in survivors (Op den Velde et al. 1993). However, the impact of these works on psychiatry as a whole was rather low. It was Vietnam and not World War II that lured many psychiatrists into entering the complicated but intriguing and challenging field of psychic trauma.

By now, it has become apparent that survivors who have hitherto been able to cope adequately with their traumatic experiences may suffer from a worsening or late onset of posttraumatic complaints during the later phases of the life cycle. Already in 1946, Tas—a survivor himself—predicted the possibility of a delayed onset of posttraumatic reactions in survivors of Nazi-persecution. Indeed, a symptom-free interval in World War II survivors has been described by various authors (Bastiaans 1957; Krystal 1968). At first, the interest of researchers and clinicians alike was primarily focused on clarifications of the so-called latency period. It was obvious that the mental health professionals concerned found it hard to understand that such horrifying and severe traumata could be endured without severe and persistent psychic damage. To explain this latency period, most authors pointed to divergent coping or defense mechanisms, such as denial and repression, or strong reaction formations, like a rigid concentration on external matters and occupational achievements. It is a sad fact that sometimes after more than four decades of successful adjustment, posttraumatic symptomatology still can emerge.

Only recently, the question arose, what could be possible causes for a recurrence or exacerbation of posttraumatic symptoms. It was found that in many instances the end of the symptom-free interval coincided with the transition of middle to late adulthood. In 1981, the *Journal of Geriatric Psychiatry* devoted a special issue to the fate of aging survivors of persecution. The late onset or worsening of posttraumatic symptomatology is often explained as a consequence of a gradual deterioration of coping mechanisms caused by the decline of physical and mental strength while getting old. It is generally believed that the particular stresses of middle and late life can trigger posttraumatic symptoms. Others highlight the importance of external events, like the threat of a new war in periods of socioeconomic and political tension and instability. There is, for instance, clinical evidence that the 1991 Gulf War served as a trigger for an acute manifestation of PTSD in some survivors of World War II (Musaph 1991; Shatan 1991). Life events that somehow resemble or symbolize past traumatic experiences may cause an exacerbation or sudden onset of symptoms.

Several recent studies, including the present one, indicate that elderly survivors of World War II are at risk for a tardive onset of posttraumatic reactions. In various geriatric institutions in the United States, it has been observed that elderly survivors of Nazi-persecution suffer from increased vulnerability to the stresses that go hand in hand with the process of aging (Honigman-Cooper 1979). In a study of 100 Dutch World War II survivors who applied for compensation, Kuilman and Suttorp (1989) found a majority of subjects in which a late onset or worsening of symptomatology during midlife and old age had taken place. They concluded that the delayed onset was often precipitated by life events. Of all patients, 43% reported meaningful life events 1 year prior to exacerbation. Occupational problems (25%), wherein the loss of a job was the main problem for 19%, was followed in frequency (20%) by a confrontation with the loss of, or separation from, nearest relatives. A study by Lomranz et al. (1985) with a nonclinical population of aging Holocaust survivors in Israel showed that survivors were more past-oriented and generally more pessimistic in their attitudes toward life events than the control group. Furthermore, their experiences during the persecution played an intense and significant role in their time orientation and reminiscences. However, it has not become clear whether this specific time orientation of elderly survivors had developed during the process of aging or (much) earlier in the course of their lives.

In a study of 86 elderly Holocaust survivors in Israel, Robinson et al. (1990) reported that although the survivors had been, and still were, quite capable to cope and adjust, many appeared to suffer from various posttraumatic symptoms. In their nonclinical sample, 60% suffered from physical illnesses connected to experiences during persecution; 75% suffered from one or more symptoms of the survivor syndrome, such as paroxysmal hypermnesia, depressive moods, nightmares, neurasthenia, and anxiety, since the end of the war with fluctuating severity to date.

Indeed, it is mainly from the survivors of Nazi-persecution

that mental health professionals learned of a possible delayed onset of posttraumatic pathology. Most studies about the nature, incidence, and course of posttraumatic disorders in World War II victims concern Jewish Holocaust survivors, concentration camp survivors, prisoners of war, and military veterans (Op den Velde et al. 1993). However, in the occupied European countries, large-scale civilian resistance to the German occupiers was carried out. In scientific research, resistance veterans are an almost forgotten group of war victims.

Stress as a Consequence of Participation in the Resistance

In May 1940, the Netherlands were invaded by the German Army. The badly equipped Dutch forces had to capitulate 5 days later. At the beginning of the military occupation, the Nazis allowed daily life to continue fairly normally. The imprisoned Dutch military were released. In the course of 1940, however, the persecution and deportation of the Jewish community began to take shape. The Dutch population reacted with growing aversion. Strikes resulted, which marked the beginning of large-scale resistance to the German occupier. Gradually, Dutch industry and agriculture were abused to support the German war efforts. In the Netherlands, this meant an increasing shortage of food and coal for heating, which eventually culminated in widespread urban famine in the winter of 1944–1945. More damaging to the Dutch was perhaps the gradual Nazi-infiltration in important sectors of administration and the police forces. This meant that the Germans had full access to all kinds of data on the Dutch population. Jews, and all those suspected of anti-Nazi sympathies, were removed from their positions and replaced by others of less "suspicious" backgrounds.

Resistance took a variety of forms, such as aid to persons living in hiding, including members of the Allied Air Forces that crashed over occupied territory. News reporting was also an important activity. The press and radio were censored by the Nazis, and numerous illegal news bulletins were printed and distributed. On a more modest scale, espionage and armed actions were carried out. In 1944, an underground army was organized and trained. The primary tasks of this hidden army were to assist the advancing Allied troops and to secure law enforcement after the expected retreat of the German troops.

Those who were active in the resistance movements were very heterogeneous (Warmbrunn 1963). Young and old, men and women, the healthy and infirm, they all did their part. The Dutch population (8.9 million people) was in fact divided into three parts. Approximately 4% were sympathetic toward the German occupier and national-socialism; some estimated 2% offered active resistance; and there also was the silent majority who in general strongly disapproved of the Nazi rule but lacked the courage to risk their lives. The people tried to live their lives as much as they were used to, and many were blind or indifferent to the extensive suffering around them.

In the immediate postwar period, people hardly gave themselves time to reflect on the previous period, or to deal with their emotions. The disorganized and plundered country claimed all available energy for its reconstruction and recovery. Collectively as well as individually, one tried to forget the years of German occupation as soon as possible. The care for disabled military veterans and concentration camp survivors was based on the principle of rest and good food. Psychological problems were seen as a temporary burden that would vanish spontaneously. This general attitude hindered adequate mastering of traumatic war experiences.

By now, it is generally known that participation in resistance movements was extremely stressful. Active resisters had to cope with various stressful experiences. First of all, there was the tension of the resistance work itself. There was no escape from the knowledge that one's life and the lives of one's family were constantly endangered. In addition to this was the perpetual fear of being betrayed. Those who sympathized with the Nazis—the so-called Quislings—often acted as informers for the German Secret Police (the "Gestapo").

Because of betrayal, carelessness, or sheer bad luck, many resistance participants were arrested. This was often followed by cruel interrogations, sustained periods of solitary confinement, and other forms of torture. The fear of "spilling the beans" and feelings of insecurity were tormenting. Subsequently, they were executed or imprisoned in labor camps, prisons, or concentration camps. In particular in the concentration camps, the conditions were extremely poor. Hard labor, frequent beatings, bad nutrition, insufficient protection against the cold, and lack of medical care were the common fate of the inmates. Many also suffered from the powerlessness that they experienced by seeing fellow prisoners being hung or beaten to death before their eyes. The hardships of the concentration camps are reflected by the mortality figures. In particular for the elderly, the chance of survival was minimal. At the Dachau concentration camp, for example, the mortality rate was 100% for Dutch male prisoners over the age of 57 compared with only 18% for those ages 27–31 (Leliefeld and Van Staden ten Brink 1982).

A Study of Elderly Dutch Resistance Veterans

In 1985, the "Stichting 1940–1945," a Dutch foundation that promotes the material and immaterial interests of former resistance participants and their next of kin, initiated a study on the mental and physical well-being of resistance veterans.

A nonclinical sample of 147 male resistance veterans was studied. They were all born been January 1, 1920, and January 1, 1926. During World War II they were between 15 and 25 years old. The sample is not representative for all male resistance veterans because they all applied for a special disability pension. As a consequence of their applying for this pension, their experiences during the war (e.g., the actual duration of their participation in the resistance and, for many, the time spent in German prisons and concentration camps) were documented in detail and impartially verified (Op den Velde et al. 1993).

All of these 147 subjects were interviewed at home by trained interviewers. The subjects, furthermore, completed a series of questionnaires, measuring PTSD, depression, insomnia, anxiety, anger, and vital exhaustion (Op den Velde et al. 1990, 1991, 1993). Some sociodemographic characteristics and the war experiences of the veterans are summarized in Table 4–1 and Table 4–2. In a subsample of 30 subjects, sleeping problems were studied by means of continuous ambulatory sleep-wake polygraphic recordings (De Groen et al. 1992).

Results

PTSD

The prevalence of PTSD as defined by DSM-III-R (American Psychiatric Association 1987) proved to be high in these elderly resistance veterans; 56% suffered from current PTSD, and in 34% PTSD in partial remission was found. In fact, only less than 4% of these veterans never had had any symptom of

Table 4–1. Some sociodemographic characteristics of 147 male Dutch resistance veterans in a nonclinical sample

Characteristic	Percentage
Highest completed level of education	
Primary school	36.7
Vocational training	27.9
High school	29.3
University	6.1
Marital status	
Currently married	68.7
Widowed	9.5
Never married	2.1
Divorced	19.7

PTSD (Hovens et al. 1992). Because all subjects were granted a special war disability pension, these figures most probably do not represent the prevalence of PTSD in the entire group of resistance veterans. In an additional study of two nonclinical samples of resistance veterans who never applied for a disability pension, ages 60–65 years, a substantially lower incidence of PTSD was found as measured on a self-rating scale (see Table 4–3) (Hovens et al. 1994).

However, the intensity of the PTSD symptoms appears to be highly variable. This was rated by the interviewers on a 5-point scale (Table 4–4). Some of the subjects with "mild" or "moderate" PTSD symptoms according to the interviewers did not fulfill all the DSM-III criteria for PTSD (e.g., symptoms from criteria B, C, and D). Therefore they are listed in Table 4–3 under "no current PTSD."

The onset of the first symptoms of PTSD was also highly variable. Several resistance veterans reported apparently symptom-free intervals of many years (see Table 4–5).

In about 50% of these veterans, PTSD became manifest only more than 20 years after the end of World War II.

Table 4–2.   War experiences of 147 resistance veterans in a nonclinical sample

Length of imprisonment (months)	Period of resistance participation (%) ($N = 73$)	Duration of concentration camp imprisonment following resistance participation (%) ($N = 74$)
No imprisonment		49.1
0–6	9.4	12.3
7–12	14.0	15.7
13–24	27.2	9.6
25–36	15.6	8.2
37–48	10.3	4.8
49–60	23.5	0

Vital Exhaustion

"Vital exhaustion" is increasingly recognized as an important behavioral risk factor in near-future myocardial infarction and sudden cardiac death patients (Appels and Mulder 1988). It has been defined as a state characterized by feelings of increased irritability, unusual tiredness, and general malaise (Falger et al. 1988). This state occurs most commonly among those who are faced with a life crisis or with a prolonged period of work overload. The state may be transient but, in interaction with already existing somatic deteriorations, it may contribute to the onset of disease, in particular myocardial infarction and sudden cardiac death. So far, vital exhaustion has been primarily studied as a risk indicator for coronary heart

Table 4–3.   Comparison of the prevalence of posttraumatic stress disorder (PTSD) in three nonclinical samples of Dutch resistance veterans, ages 60–65 years

	Disability pension (%)	No disability pension (%)	
	Men ($N = 147$)	Men ($N = 680$)	Women ($N = 144$)
Current PTSD	56.0	27.4	20.1
No current PTSD	44.0	72.6	79.9

Table 4–4.   Overall impression of the interviewers of the intensity of the symptoms of posttraumatic stress disorder (PTSD) in a nonclinical sample of 147 male resistance veterans

Intensity	N	%
No PTSD symptoms	48	32.5
Mild symptoms	27	18.3
Moderate symptoms	30	20.4
Severe symptoms	35	23.8
Very severe symptoms	7	4.8

disease. In these patients, vital exhaustion appeared to be associated with angina pectoris, type A coronary-prone behavior, chronic exposure to life crises, excessive smoking and coffee consumption, and sleep complaints. The conceptual parallels with chronic PTSD are intuitively appealing. Therefore, the relationships between PTSD, vital exhaustion, and a number of coronary heart disease risk indicators were studied in the first nonclinical sample of resistance veterans. Vital exhaustion was measured by a 21-item self-report rating scale, the Maastricht Questionnaire (Falger and Op den Velde 1991; Falger et al. 1992).

Veterans with current PTSD reported vital exhaustion to a significantly larger extent than veterans without current PTSD (see Table 4–6). However, there appears to be a considerable overlap between some of the symptoms of PTSD and signs of vital exhaustion. To gain insight into the aspects of vital exhaustion that were associated with current PTSD, an item analysis was performed. All 21 items discriminated positively between PTSD and non-PTSD veterans. Moreover, 13 of these items did not represent DSM-III-R criteria for PTSD. When only the latter items were studied, the difference between PTSD and non-PTSD veterans was still highly significant. During the interviews about PTSD, data about previous myocardial infarction, angina pectoris, hypertension, type A/B personality, and current smoking were collected as well. These

Table 4–5. Onset of first symptoms of posttraumatic stress disorder in a nonclinical sample of 147 male resistance veterans

Time period	N	%
1945–1950	39	26
1951–1960	12	8
1961–1970	30	20
1971–1980	35	24
1981–1988	9	6
Unclear	22	15

Table 4–6. Vital exhaustion and coronary risk factors in a nonclinical sample of resistance veterans and same-age comparison groups

	Resistance veterans			Coronary cases (N = 65)	Hospital control subjects (N = 79)
Risk factors	All (N = 147)	PTSD (N = 82)	No PTSD (N = 56)		
Mean age (years)	64.1	63.8	64.5	61.3	61.0
Mean vital exhaustion score	23.6	30.1	15.5	17.9	12.9
Prior myocardial infarction (%)	**9**	**9**	**10**	**100**	
Current angina pectoris (%)	26	31	14	26	7
Type A behavior pattern (%)	73	82	63	60	51
Current smoking (%)	51	57	34	82	60

PTSD = posttraumatic stress

data were compared with a different study in same-age male heart patients and hospital control subjects. The latter had never suffered a myocardial infarction.

Veterans with PTSD showed significantly more current angina pectoris, smoked more frequently, and were more often assessed as type A than veterans without current PTSD. They also scored higher on vital exhaustion. When compared with recent coronary patients, resistance veterans were more often considered type A, and they were also characterized as being exhausted to an unusual extent. Thus, type A behavior may very well be associated with the development of PTSD and may promote a state of vital exhaustion. Furthermore, vital exhaustion may be considered as a long-term outcome of exposure to severe wartime trauma. This exhaustion appears to reflect a state of "loss of vital energy" and "demoralization," which is not included in PTSD as defined by DSM-III-R. Because those vitally exhausted with type A behavior, in particular, appear to be at a more than 11-fold elevated risk for a first myocardial infarction compared with same-age healthy subjects, the presently observed confluence of type A behavior, vital exhaustion, and current PTSD may indicate a high vulnerability for coronary disease in elderly patients suffering from PTSD.

Sleep Disturbances

Disturbed sleeping is one of the most frequent complaints of patients suffering from PTSD. A polysomnographic study of 30 male resistance veterans, ages 60–65 years, was carried out. Sleep studies were done at home by means of a 24-hour portable recording system (De Groen et al. 1992). The subjects were instructed to continue their daily activities as much as possible during the registration. We found in subjects with current PTSD a decrease of total sleep time, sleep efficiency, rapid eye movement (REM)-sleep latency, and deep sleep (stages III–IV).

In subjects with a high incidence of nightmares, the circadian temperature minimum and REM sleep half-time appeared to occur significantly earlier with respect to sleep onset (De Groen et al. 1990, 1992). Furthermore, a significant association was found between snoring and the occurrence of anxiety dreams (De Groen et al. 1993). Incidence of anxiety dreams was highest when snoring was accompanied by respiratory pauses.

The observed desynchronization of REM and non-REM sleep offers support for the hypothesis of inappropriate REM sleep recruitment as a generator of posttraumatic nightmares. Hypercapnia and autonomic-vegetative arousal, resulting from obstructive sleep apneic episodes in heavy snoring, may further facilitate the occurrence of nightmares in elderly subjects suffering from PTSD.

Somatic Morbidity

The prevalence of other somatic complaints and problems was also studied. The resistance veterans reported substantially more somatic complaints as compared with same-age control groups from the general population (Op den Velde et al. 1991). This enhanced number of complaints concerned all kinds of diagnoses and was not due to particular diseases.

Biographical Interviews

The general impression of the life history interviews warrants the conclusion that severe traumatic experiences and subsequent PTSD do not preclude good or even excellent social and occupational functioning for considerable periods of time. However, most of the 147 veterans did retire or were granted a disability pension at the age of 50–55 years. At the time of the study, only 6 of the 147 veterans were still partially employed. The mean year of retirement was 1975 (± 7.33) (Op den Velde et al. 1991). Problems and conflicts with colleagues at work often promoted early retirement. During the interviews, it became clear that, in particular, manifestations of vital exhaustion, chronic fatigue, insomnia, and irritability forced them to terminate their occupational careers. It was often observed that symptoms of PTSD and of vital exhaustion not only continued but sometimes even grew worse after retirement and after their special disability pension had been granted. Most veterans stated that the loss of work was a burden, which exerted unexpected negative effects on their coping with their traumatic war past. A similar pattern was observed in Scandinavian war sailors (Hartvig 1977).

More than ever before, the resistance veterans experienced painful reminiscences related to their war experiences. From the middle-age transition onward, they seriously contemplated on the meaning of life as they looked back on their previous life episodes. They became occupied once again with questions about the sense of their resistance deeds, the risks they personally took, and the endangering of others. Also, they compulsively asked themselves whether the suffering and sacrifice of their deceased resistance comrades had been worthwhile or could have been avoided. Apparently, the phase of the trauma recovery process that requires the placing of traumatic experiences in a new, more acceptable and meaningful frame of reference has been reached but not worked through. In general, these veterans were reluctant to share their feelings with others, even with their closest relatives. They have the idea that it is a sign of weakness of character, or even of insanity, to have this kind of reminiscence so many years after the end of World War II. They further stick to the belief that they have to protect others from their painful memories, doubts, and fears. Relatives and friends sometimes suspect that awful war memories play a role in their behavior, but consider it wise not to evoke more emotions by bringing up the war for discussion. Therefore these veterans are caught in a conspiracy of silence, which may lead to depression, shame, self-reproach, and finally withdrawal in utmost disappointment (see Danieli 1993).

Discussion

The burdens and losses of the later phases of the life span are not scarce and not easy to overcome. One's decreasing physical and mental abilities, the confrontation with the death of friends and relatives and with one's own future death are in themselves difficult enough to cope with. But many other kinds of losses, too, will have to be faced during the later phases of life, such as the loss of responsibilities, of independence, and of one's previous position in society. These losses usually occur gradually, once the age of retirement is reached, and they mostly coincide with the time that one's children come of age and leave the parental home.

As mentioned earlier, the delayed onset of posttraumatic symptomatology in elderly survivors is often explained as a consequence of the confrontation during the transmission of middle to late life with physical decline and illness, with hospitalization, and with—this time—inescapable death, which triggers recollections of similar unworked-through experiences during the war. Although survivors of trauma are sometimes able to cope with the stresses of old age, it has been observed that some survivors give up entirely and surrender completely to inactivity, to a pessimistic view of their past and future, and to a lack of meaning of their vicissitudes during World War II.

In victims of Nazi-persecution, the difficulties encountered during the process of aging can be particularly hard to tackle. It has been observed by clinicians that it is not uncommon for strong feelings about lost loved ones to emerge at the end of a survivor's life, thereby expressing pent-up longing, guilt, and depression (Kahana 1981). Also, the separation from children who leave the parental home is often extremely painful for survivors who have lost so many of their relatives and friends during World War II. Resistance veterans, as a special group of trauma survivors, have encountered many losses too. Many comrades were captured or killed in action. Uncompleted grief, but also guilt feelings, may be reactivated by the losses of friends and relatives during old age.

Kahana (1981) observed a late onset of posttraumatic symptomatology, paradoxically, when survivors finally succeeded in establishing a normal existence. The then diminished need for energy caused a breakdown of defensive reaction formations. In this regard, the high incidence of vital exhaustion that was found in our sample, also in veterans without current PTSD, is certainly not without meaning. The repression of memories and affects and coping with everyday life demand much of the energy of the traumatized individual. When these vital energies flow away during the process of aging, the hitherto adequate repressive and coping mechanisms may fail (Davidson 1987; Krystal 1981).

Reaching the age of retirement could be particularly difficult for the present population. Although in many subjects in the past the focus of attention was primarily directed on occupational and economical achievements, self-esteem was mainly derived from the ability to work hard and from occupational status. In addition, the distraction that was offered by social contacts at work disappears by losing the contacts with former colleagues, and this may well cause social isolation in the elderly survivor. In resistance veterans, the societal conspiracy of silence, as has been explained, had already given them a sense of isolation from others.

Memories, manifest or latent, play an important role in the process of aging. As Coleman (1986) pointed out, reminiscence during old age in general need not necessarily be judged negatively, as was customary until recently in gerontological thought. The modern "life-span perspective" on the process of aging has learned that the function and quality of reminiscence in old age is closely related to each individual life history. In traumatized subjects, however, memories can be thrusting and intrusive, and efforts are made to ward these off, whereas in others a nearly compulsive tendency to ruminate on past events can be present (Coleman 1986). There is evidence that traumatized subjects are more vulnerable to be tortured by their formerly suppressed trauma-related memories during the process of aging. In the study of Robinson et al. (1990), with a nonclinical sample of Holocaust survivors, 82% of the subjects reported sudden attacks of painful memories of traumatic events. In their study, of all symptoms of the survivor syndrome, hypermnesia scored highest. In another study by Hertz (1990), comparing reminiscences and nostalgic feelings in two groups of elderly immigrants in Israel, the Holocaust survivors were more prone to reminiscences in the later years of their lives than those who had not been threatened with physical and mental annihilation, but had also been exposed to powerful environmental stresses as a consequence of migration.

According to Cath (1981), an important task of each aging individual is the maintenance of self-coherence and self-continuity. People who as a consequence of traumatization already have difficulties in feeling cohesive, experience these difficulties more urgently when they reach the last phases of the life span. Old age is the final stage in the life cycle. The word *cycle* indicates that life is generally perceived as a continuing line— although shaped to form a circle. Massive trauma, however, means a rupture in the life cycle. As such it is a fierce and often successful attack on psychic integrity. As a result, the awareness of the "self" is split into a pretraumatic self, a traumatic self, and a posttraumatic self (Laufer 1988). The integration of these three selves is a hard task to accomplish. Amnesia for the pretraumatic self or an idealization of that particular period of life, as is often seen in victims of persecution, can be understood as an effort of the individual to deny the rupture in one's life and to establish a sense of continuity between the former self and the posttraumatic self. However, because the traumatic self is mostly looked on with awe, shame, and anger, the accompanying memories and affects are strongly repressed. The integration of the three selves can be accomplished only when these negative affects can be faced and the loss of the previous self can be mourned for. In old age, grief is more or less inherent as a consequence of the many losses that accompany it. Thus, mourning is also part and parcel of adequate adaptation to aging. Especially in old age, the acceptance and integration of past and present states demand mourning. However, the capacity to mourn in survivors of trauma is often impaired. Krystal (1981) stressed that posttraumatic states are characterized by affect intolerance. Others hold an incapacity to mourn for the main pathogenic factor in the etiology of the survivor syndrome (Grubrich-Simitis 1979; Meerloo 1968). To be able to mourn, however, a certain amount of affect tolerance is required. Furthermore, the mourning for previous, analogous losses is rarely completed in severely traumatized people, and the new losses may well trigger suppressed and postponed grief.

The disintegrating effects of psychic trauma can be reduced or undone only when sufficient mourning has taken place and when acceptance of one's fate and a new sense of self-coherence and continuity have been achieved. If the completion of the life cycle is indeed the main task of old age, it is obvious that traumatized people—who have not been able to work through their experiences and who encounter problems during old age that resemble and symbolize these experiences—are severely hindered to do so. In addition, however, intrusive reminiscences of the traumatic past can be hindrances in the mourning processes. Experiencing insomnia, vital exhaustion, anxiety, and depression can be additional burdens for mourning in the elderly.

It can be concluded that there is a mutual reinforcement of the specific burdens of the later phases of the life span, which can result in PTSD in elderly survivors of war trauma. The commonalities between the process of aging and the effects of psychic trauma may well have been the reason that "premature aging" (Fédération Internationale des Résistants 1973; Schenck 1977; Thygesen and Hermann 1954) was among the first symptoms generally recognized in survivors of persecution. Apparently, the essentially invalidating and degenerating effects of psychic trauma on human physical and mental integrity have been intuitively understood, before the etiology and pathogenesis of posttraumatic symptomatology were described in more psychodynamic terms.

Summary

Dutch resistance veterans show a high incidence of PTSD. Even more than 45 years after World War II, 34.5% of the population under study suffered from current PTSD (see Table 4–3). The observation in this study of a delayed onset or reoccurrence of PTSD (see Table 4–5) in World War II resistance veterans during the transition of middle to late life is not rare at all. The onset of posttraumatic symptomatology frequently coincides with an enforced inactivity during middle and late life. This inactivity is mostly caused by the loss of work, a separation from relatives, or by illness.

Sleep architecture is disturbed in elderly resistance veterans. A desynchronization of REM- and non-REM sleep was found. Obstructive sleep apnea, a far from rare condition in the elderly, may facilitate the occurrence of posttraumatic nightmares.

Subjects with current PTSD suffered significantly more from vital exhaustion and were more often of type A behavior than the non-PTSD group. This may imply that elderly resistance veterans with current PTSD are at risk for coronary diseases.

From the results of these studies, we may expect that other groups, such as Vietnam veterans, will be at risk for a worsening or sudden onset of posttraumatic symptomatology during the later phases of their lives.

References

American Psychiatric Association: Diagnostic and Statistical Manual of Mental Disorders, 3rd Edition. Washington, DC, American Psychiatric Association, 1980

American Psychiatric Association: Diagnostic and Statistical Manual of Mental Disorders, 3rd Edition, Revised. Washington, DC, American Psychiatric Association, 1987

Appels A, Mulder P: Excess fatigue as a precursor of myocardial infarction. Eur Heart J 9:758–764, 1988

Bastiaans J: Psychosomatische gevolgen van onderdrukking en verzet [Psychosomatic consequences of oppression and resistance]. Dissertation, University of Amsterdam, Netherlands, 1957

Bastiaans J: The KZ-syndrome: a thirty year study of the effects on victims of Nazi concentration camps. Revue Medico-Chirurgicale de Jassy 78:573–578, 1974

Cath SH: The aging survivor: the effects of the Holocaust on life-cycle experiences: the creation and recreation of families. J Geriatr Psychiatry 14:155–163, 1981

Coleman PG: Ageing and Reminiscence Processes: Social and Clinical Implications. New York, Wiley, 1986

Danieli Y: Diagnostic and therapeutic use of the multigenerational family tree on working with survivors and children of survivors of the Nazi Holocaust, in International Handbook of Traumatic Stress Syndromes. Edited by Wilson JP, Rafael B. New York, Plenum, 1993, pp 889–898

Davidson S: Trauma in the life cycle of the individual and the collective consciousness in relation to war and persecution, in Society and Trauma of War (Sinaï Series No 4). Edited by Dasberg H, Davidson S, Durlacher GL. Assen, Netherlands, Van Gorcum 1987, pp 14–32

De Groen JHM, Op den Velde W, Van Duijn H, et al: Posttraumatic nightmares and timing of REM sleep. Journal of Interdisciplinary Cycle Research 21:192–193, 1990

De Groen JHM, Op den Velde W, Van Duijn H: Posttraumatic nightmares and timing of REM sleep, in Chronobiology and Chronomedicine. Edited by Diez-Noguera A, Cambras T. Frankfurt am Main, Germany, P Lang, 1992, pp 259–261

De Groen JHM, Op den Velde W, Hovens JE, et al: Snoring and anxiety dreams. Sleep 16:35–36, 1993

Eitinger L: Pathology of the concentration camp syndrome. Arch Gen Psychiatry 5:371–379, 1961

Falger PRJ, Op den Velde W: Long-term health consequences of being a World War II resistance veteran: posttraumatic stress disorder and cardiovascular disease (abstract). Psychosom Med 53:226, 1991

Falger P, Schouten E, Appels A: Sleep complaints, behavioral characteristics and vital exhaustion in myocardial infarction cases. Psychology and Health 2:231–258, 1988

Falger PRJ, Op den Velde W, Hovens JE, et al: Current posttraumatic stress disorder, "vital exhaustion," and cardiovascular morbidity in male Dutch resistance veterans of World War II. Psychother Psychosom 57:164–171, 1992

Fédération Internationale des Résistants (eds): Ermüdung und vorzeitiges Altern: Folge von Extrembelastungen [Exhaustion and premature aging]. Leipzig, Germany, Kommissionsverlag JA Barth, 1973

Grubrich-Simitis I: Extremtraumatizierung als kummulatives Trauma [Extreme trauma as cumulative trauma]. Psyche 33:991–1023, 1979

Hartvig P: Krigsseilerssyndromet [The war-sailor syndrome]. Nordisk Psykiatrisk Tidsskrift 29:302–312, 1977

Hertz DG: Trauma and nostalgia: new aspects on the coping of ageing Holocaust survivors. Isr J Psychiatry Relat Sci 27:189–198, 1990

Honigman-Cooper R: Concentration camp survivors: a challenge for geriatric nursing. Nurs Clin North Am 14:621–628, 1979

Hovens JE, Falger PRJ, Op den Velde W, et al: Occurrence of posttraumatic stress disorder among Dutch World War II resistance veterans according to the SCID. Journal of Anxiety Disorders 6:147–157, 1992

Hovens JE, Falger PRJ, Op den Velde W, et al: PTSD in Dutch resistance veterans from World War II in relation to trait anxiety and depression. Psychol Rep 74:275–285, 1994

Kahana RJ: The aging survivor of the Holocaust: discussion: reconciliation between the generations: a last chance. J Geriatr Psychiatry 14:225–289, 1981

Kardiner A: The Traumatic Neuroses of War. New York, Paul Hoeber, 1941

Krystal H (ed): Massive Psychic Trauma. New York, Little, Brown, 1968

Krystal H: The aging survivor of the Holocaust: integration and self-healing in posttraumatic states. J Geriatr Psychiatry 14:165–189, 1981

Kuilman M, Suttorp O: Late onset posttraumatic spectrum disorders in survivors of Nazi-terror: a retrospective study of 100 patients (1973–1988). Paper read at the Congress "Psychische Schäden alternder Überlebenden des Nazi-Terrors und ihrer Nachkomen." Hannover, Federal Republic of Germany, 11–14 October, 1989

Laufer RS: The serial self: war trauma, identity and adult development, in Human Adaptation to Extreme Stress From the Holocaust to Vietnam. Edited by Wilson JP, Harel Z, Kahana B. New York, Plenum, 1988, pp 33–53

Leliefeld H, Van Staden ten Brink A: Dutch Prisoners of the Concentration Camp Dachau 1941–1979: a Study of Mortality and Causes of Death. Alphen a/d Ryn, Netherlands, Samson/Sijthoff, 1982

Lomranz J, Shmotkin D, Zechovoy A, et al: Time orientation in Nazi concentration camp survivors: forty years after. Am J Orthopsychiatry 55:230–236, 1985

Maugham S: Points of View. Garden City, NY, Doubleday, 1959

Meerloo JAM: Delayed mourning in victims of extermination camps, in Massive Psychic Trauma. Edited by Krystal H. New York, Little, Brown, 1968, pp 72–74

Musaph H: De Golfoorlog als trigger voor een late post-traumatische stress-reactie [The Gulf War as a trigger for late onset PTSD]. Tijdschrift voor Psychotherapie 19:356–361, 1991

Op den Velde W, Falger PRJ, De Groen JHM, et al: Current psychiatric complaints of Dutch resistance veterans: a feasibility study. Journal of Traumatic Stress 3:351–358, 1990

Op den Velde W, Falger PRJ, Hovens JE, et al: De psychische en lichamelijke klachten van verzetsdeelnemers [Psychiatric and somatic complaints of Resistance veterans]. Jaarboek Psychiatrie Psychotherapie 3:96–110, 1991

Op den Velde W, Hovens JE, Falger PRJ, et al: PTSD in Dutch resistance veterans from World War II, in International Handbook of Traumatic Stress Syndromes. Edited by Wilson JP, Raphael B. New York, Plenum, 1993, pp 219–230

Robinson S, Rapaport J, Durst R, et al: The late effects of Nazi-persecution among elderly Holocaust survivors. Acta Psychiatr Scand 82:311–315, 1990

Schenck EG: Voralterung als Folge exogener Einflüsse auf eine endogene Bereitschaft [Premature aging as a consequence of external influences]. Therapie der Gegenwart 166:446–470, 1977

Shatan CF: The Gulf—50 year gap in onset of PTSD. Proceedings of the 7th Annual Convention of the Society for Traumatic Stress Studies, Washington, DC, October 24–27, 1991, p 11

Tas J: Psychische stoornissen in concentratiekampen en bij teruggekeerden [Psychic disorders in concentration camps and in those who survived]. Maandblad Geestelijke Volksgezondheid 6:143–150, 1946

Thygesen P, Hermann K: La déportation dans les camps de concentration allemands et ses séquelles. Edited by the Fédération Internationale des Résistants. Paris, France, Fédération Internationale des Résistants, 1954

Venzlaff U: Mental disorders resulting from racial persecution outside of concentration camps. Int J Soc Psychiatry 4:177–183, 1964

Warmbrunn W: The Dutch Under German Occupation 1940–1945. Stanford, CA, Stanford University Press, 1963

Part II

Late-Age Trauma

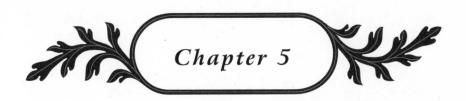

Chapter 5

Severe Stress and the Elderly

Are Older Adults at Increased Risk for Posttraumatic Stress Disorder?

Robert B. Fields, Ph.D.

I n this chapter, the hypothesis that older adults are at greater risk than younger adults for the development of psychiatric problems following exposure to a traumatic experience is addressed. In general terms, the construct of risk, or vulnerability, has been used to conceptualize the etiology of several psychiatric conditions (e.g., schizophrenia—see Zubin and Spring 1977). An individual is at risk, or vulnerable, for a particular disorder if the likelihood that he or she will meet diagnostic criteria for that disorder is greater than the population at large. Studies designed to test vulnerability hypotheses typically involve attempts to identify characteristics of specific "at risk" individuals that differentiate them from those who are not at risk. Although many such studies focus on genetic or environmental factors, others explore the role that demographic variables (e.g., age) may play in contributing to an individual's at-risk status.

With regard to posttraumatic psychiatric syndromes, an age-related "differential vulnerability" hypothesis implies that exposure to trauma produces negative effects on psychosocial functioning in the elderly and that these effects are greater in older adults than they are in younger adults. It also implies that this age effect occurs independent of the type or severity of trauma experienced. Thus, the differential vulnerability hypothesis could be tested by assessing the rates of general psychiatric and specific trauma-related symptomatology in the following comparison groups: the elderly exposed to traumatic experiences of different types and severities, matched elderly not exposed to trauma, and younger adults exposed to the same traumatic events as the older adults.

Not surprisingly, no studies exist that comprehensively address all aspects of this hypothesis, and only a limited number have systematically investigated the role of age in determining outcome following traumatic exposure. When testing the differential vulnerability hypothesis, the issue of the type of trauma experienced is an important one for a variety of reasons. Some experiences (e.g., combat) are less frequent among older adults and as a result do not permit age-related comparisons. Although events such as natural disasters are less age specific, there is ample evidence that the type and severity of disaster clearly affect physical and psychological outcome. For example, several authors (Baum et al. 1983; Bolin 1988; Frederick 1980; Green 1991; Smith et al. 1988) have discussed differences in symptom constellation following disasters that are human-made compared with those that are the result of natural phenomena. Similarly, several studies (e.g., Phifer and Norris 1989) have suggested that symptomatology differs as a function of the severity of the disaster. The relevance of these findings to the differential vulnerability hypothesis is that even if age differences occur following one type of disaster, they may not be generalizable to another.

Another aspect of an at-risk model that is frequently overlooked are the implications for those individuals at both ends of the vulnerability continuum. It is well documented that the same stressful event does not produce the same effects in everyone who experiences it. For reasons that are becoming better understood with time, several preexisting and posttraumatic factors appear to mediate the influence of the trauma on any specific individual (McFarlane 1991). Using the example of a natural disaster, the capacity to deal with the aftermath of an event that caused personal or property loss or both and over which there was no control varies dramatically. If the trauma is sufficiently severe, most elderly are likely to experience psychological consequences (Miller et al. 1981; Phifer and Norris 1989; Shore et al. 1986). However, at the most invulnerable end of the continuum, an elderly individual may be able to go through a normal grieving process and even "grow" from the experience through his or her involvement in helping others (Bell 1978; Lyons 1991; Melick and Logue 1985–1986).

What about the other end of the continuum? If decreased vulnerability lessens the subjective impact of a traumatic experience, does increased vulnerability worsen the trauma of less-stressful events? Of particular relevance for the elderly is the possibility that once one's personal coping resources are significantly compromised, many more environmental events may cause greater than expected psychosocial consequences. For example, a cognitively impaired, socially isolated, and therefore vulnerable elderly individual may experience an unwanted move from an apartment to a nursing home as a "disaster." The extensive, and controversial, literature on environmental relocation in the elderly includes numerous reports of negative effects on well-being but has not yet considered these negative effects from a posttraumatic stress disorder (PTSD) perspective.

In this chapter, literature relevant to the question of whether the elderly are at greater risk for negative psychiatric and psychosocial consequences following traumatic events is reviewed. Studies addressing the prevalence of PTSD and other related psychiatric disorders as a function of age are discussed. General psychosocial and psychiatric response follow-ing natural disasters is also discussed as a means of broadening PTSD models to test the differential vulnerability hypothesis. Finally, the possible utility of a PTSD framework for under-standing the literature on involuntary relocation of the elderly is reviewed.

Epidemiology of PTSD Among Older Adults

Remarkably little is know about the prevalence and phenome-nology of PTSD among older adults. In two published reviews of geriatric psychiatry (Busse and Blazer 1989; Sadavoy et al. 1991), no reference to PTSD appears despite the fact that these volumes contain chapters on anxiety disorders, sleep dis-orders, and the epidemiology of psychiatric disorders in the elderly. Just as surprising is the omission of any discussion of PTSD in a work devoted entirely to anxiety in the elderly (Salzman and Lebowitz 1991).

The prevalence of anxiety disorders in general appears to decline above age 65 (Abrams 1991; Brickman and Eisdorfer 1989), although this conclusion is somewhat controversial. As noted by Shamoian (1991) in his review of this literature, early studies in this area that assessed symptoms of anxiety with different measures among a variety of populations led, not sur-prisingly, to conflicting results. Some studies noted an increase in anxiety symptoms with age (Gaitz and Scott 1972; Warheit et al. 1986), whereas others reported no difference (Leighton et al. 1963), and still others observed fewer anxiety symptoms with age (Magni and DeLeo 1984). More recent studies have utilized structured diagnostic interviews with larger, typically community-dwelling, elderly samples. Based on the Epidemio-logic Catchment Area (ECA) study, Regier et al. (1988) reported a decline with age in the 1-month prevalence rates of anxiety disorders. Among the elderly group, women met crite-ria for an anxiety disorder approximately twice as often as men.

Phobia was the most common anxiety disorder reported for both sexes. Six-month and lifetime prevalence rates of anxiety disorders were also noted to be less among the elderly (Blazer et al. 1991; Brickman and Eisdorfer 1989).

Focusing on generalized anxiety disorder in particular, Blazer et al. (1991) reported that the age at onset of this disorder was relatively stable between ages 18 and 64, with a dramatic drop-off above age 65. The correlation between these data and PTSD is unknown. However, the fact that the elderly in general do not appear to be differentially vulnerable to anxiety disorders is relevant to the hypothesis discussed in this chapter.

Regarding PTSD, the relatively few epidemiological studies in existence have focused primarily on Vietnam veterans. Although estimates vary, most, if not all, of the studies have linked severity of traumatic experience to increased PTSD symptomatology. For example, the results of the National Vietnam Veterans Readjustment Study (Jordan et al. 1991) found that 15.2% of male and 8.5% of female Vietnam theater veterans met criteria for PTSD in the 6-month preinterview period, whereas the corresponding rates for male Vietnam era veterans and civilians were 2.5% and 1.2%, and for females were 1.1% and 0.3%, respectively. Several studies have provided additional but somewhat conflicting epidemiological information about PTSD in other groups. Breslau et al. (1991) explored the prevalence of PTSD in a sample of 1,007 young adults (i.e., ages 21–30) in the Detroit, Michigan, area. They found that 39.1% of their sample were exposed to at least one traumatic experience and that 23.6% of those exposed met criteria for PTSD. This 9.2% lifetime PTSD prevalence rate was notably higher than the rate of 1.1% reported by Helzer et al. (1987). From their review of 2,493 adults evaluated as part of the ECA survey, Helzer et al. reported increased rates of PTSD for civilians exposed to physical attack and Vietnam veterans who were not wounded (3.5%). The highest rates of PTSD were found among wounded Vietnam veterans (20%). As Breslau et al. (1991) pointed out, the discrepancy between overall prevalence rates may have partly been due to differences in data collection methods and the relative sizes of the trauma-exposed groups. Of relevance to this discussion is the fact that although the exposed group in the Helzer et al. study was quite small, no age differences were found between subjects with and without the diagnosis, or individual symptoms, of PTSD.

Another study that dealt more directly with the question of age and differential vulnerability to PTSD was completed with residents of two rural communities in the northwest United States (Shore et al. 1989). In this study, 1,025 adults ages 18–79 were administered structured psychiatric interviews (Diagnostic Interview Schedule), and a diagnosis of PTSD was reached when all four DSM-III (American Psychiatric Association 1980) criteria were met. Of the population sampled, 138 were known to have suffered "high-exposure" to the May 1980 Mount Saint Helens volcanic eruption and subsequent flooding in southwest Washington State (as determined by at least $5,000 loss in property or the death of a family member or close relative); 410 suffered "low-exposure," and 477 suffered no exposure.

Regarding the variable of age, as can be seen in Table 5–1, although the lifetime risk of a "posttraumatic stress reaction" was approximately 3% overall, the most vulnerable group was the 35- to 44-year-old group. In this sample, the lifetime risk for males ages 60–79 was 1.1%, whereas the lifetime risk for females ages 60–79 was 0%. In an earlier study of disorders related to Mount Saint Helens following the first year after the eruption, Shore et al. (1986) found higher rates of symptoms related to the eruption in the high-exposure group in general. Although women reported more distress than men in this study, no age differences were reported, and it was concluded that the "dose-response" pattern of increased symptoms among those with greater exposure was a consistent finding across all age groups. Thus, the limited available data on the epidemiology of PTSD, per se, are not consistent with an age-related differential vulnerability hypothesis.

Finally, another approach to assessing PTSD in the elderly has been to explore specific psychiatric patient populations that might be at risk. A number of studies have documented the frequent coexistence of PTSD with other psychiatric disorders (e.g., Sierles et al. 1983). Based on clinical observations that recent life stressors (e.g., death of a close friend) appeared to exacerbate PTSD-like symptoms in some patients admitted to a Veterans Administration geropsychiatric unit, we explored the prevalence of PTSD in this population (Rosen et al. 1989). Among World War II combat veterans who were admitted to a psychiatric hospital 40 years following their war experience and who met criteria for another DSM-III disorder, the prevalence of current PTSD was 27%, and the prevalence of past PTSD (for the 5-year postwar period) was 54%. These findings are relatively similar to those reported by Green et al. (1990), who assessed PTSD among survivors of the Buffalo Creek dam collapse in Buffalo Creek Valley, West Virginia, in February 1972, and found prevalence rates of 44% 2 years following this natural disaster and 28% 12 years later.

Table 5–1. Lifetime rates of posttraumatic stress disorder in two rural Northwest communities

	N	Age	PTSD
Men	129	18–34	4.0 ± 1.8
	141	35–44	5.2 ± 2.0
	135	45–59	$.7 \pm .7$
	110	60–79	1.1 ± 1.1
Women	146	18–34	2.3 ± 1.6
	140	35–44	7.9 ± 2.5
	115	45–59	2.1 ± 1.3
	109	60–79	0

Source. Reprinted with permission from Shore JH, Vollmer WM, Tatum EL: "Community Patterns of Post Traumatic Stress Disorders." *Journal of Nervous and Mental Disease* 177:681–685, 1989. Copyright 1989 by Williams & Wilkins.

Psychosocial Response Following Natural Disaster

There is a concern that arises when PTSD is diagnosed solely through the use of structured interviews. The interview process itself may result in the failure to acknowledge the presence of significant psychological distress in subjects who have some symptoms of PTSD, but not enough to meet diagnostic criteria. Most studies report that the prevalence rates for specific symptoms of PTSD are much greater than the prevalence rates for the full-blown disorder (Helzer et al. 1987). Furthermore, the method used to obtain information about symptomatology of PTSD may be problematic. In her review of PTSD assessment strategies following disasters, Green (1991) noted that the use of the Diagnostic Interview Schedule underestimated the prevalence of PTSD in general population samples when compared with the diagnoses of expert clinicians. Thus, by not limiting studies of outcome following trauma to individuals who meet criteria for PTSD, a great deal more might be learned about the effects of trauma in general, and the differential vulnerability hypothesis in particular. The literature on psychosocial response following natural disasters has been helpful in this regard.

Compared with combat or prisoner-of-war experiences, natural disasters are less age specific. However, comparing across disasters is difficult because of the tremendous variability in their scope and impact. As a result, the data in this area have been rather inconsistent. Earlier studies, perhaps based on somewhat ageist biases, predicted and reported increased negative consequences following disasters among the elderly (Lifton and Olson 1976; Moore and Friedsam 1959). Subsequent studies have found conflicting results (Cohen and Poulshock 1977; Huerta and Horton 1978; Kilijanek and Drabek 1979). When reviewing this literature, several points must be kept in mind. First, many studies that report outcome measures for different age groups did not specifically test the differential vulnerability hypothesis. As a result, negative (or positive) outcome among older samples may have been a result of variables not related to age; for example, older adults who live in less-adequate housing may be at greater risk for damage from floods or tornadoes because of their lower socioeconomic status rather than their age. Second, the disasters for which age data have been reported vary widely in type and severity and may not be generalizable. Third, only a handful of studies explored the role that age plays in predicting psychosocial outcome in the context of other variables.

From a historical perspective, early studies in this area supported a differential vulnerability hypothesis. For example, Friedsam (1961, 1962) concluded from his review of the literature on casualties from World War II and natural disasters that the elderly are a "special risk" group for both physical and psychosocial consequences. Several subsequent studies tested the suppositions that the increased risk among the elderly included risk factors of increased likelihood of death following a natural disaster, a distorted perception of their circumstances, and a tendency to underuse available resources. A number of studies lend support for the first factor, with increased casualty rates reported among the elderly following floods (Hutton 1976), hurricanes (Friedsam 1961), and tornadoes (Bolin and Klenow 1982–1983; Carter et al. 1989). Although factors such as decreased physical capacity, increased likelihood of being at home, and greater reluctance to heed warnings (Friedsam 1962) may be age related, others such as lack of available resources in times of crisis and greater likelihood of living in flood plains or less-sturdy houses may be more related to socioeconomic status than age (Carter et al. 1989; Kilijanek and Drabek 1979).

Regarding perception of circumstances, Friedsam (1961) suggested that the elderly perceive their losses as relatively greater than those of their neighbors. In his review of this literature, Fields (1992) concluded that there is not sufficient support for Friedsam's "relative deprivation" hypothesis. Although a few studies suggested that the elderly may experience more physical losses and may report more material losses following a disaster, the conclusions of a marked discrepancy between actual and perceived loss appeared to be exaggerated. In addition, the fact that the elderly often attach a greater significance to certain types of possessions was typically not taken into account by these studies (Kilijanek and Drabek 1979). Finally, regarding the use of available resources, a review of this literature (Fields 1992) suggests that as a group, the elderly ask less, complain less, and receive less in resources than younger-age ranges of the population. In part, this pattern appears to be due to a reluctance to accept "government handouts" (Huerta and Horton 1978; Kilijanek and Drabek 1979), although the elderly are more willing to use aid from sources such as home insurance agencies and the Red Cross or Salvation Army.

Regarding psychological response to natural disasters, the available literature does not consistently support the hypothesis that the elderly are an at-risk population. Clearly, older adults are negatively affected by exposure to traumatic experiences, and their reluctance to ask for help should be taken into account when planning postdisaster relief efforts. However, it does not appear that older adults suffer worse psychological consequences than younger adults. In fact, in several studies, elderly persons did as well or better than their younger counterparts. Studies of postdisaster outcome consistently suggest that the variables of prior symptom level and severity of stressor account for the most variance when predicting psychosocial and general response. When compared with these types of variables, the contribution of age is quite small and generally inconsistent with a differential vulnerability hypothesis.

Despite the problems inherent in comparing studies utilizing different methodologies to assess outcome following different types of natural disasters, it seems reasonable to conclude that most disasters are events of sufficient magnitude to produce at least short-term consequences in elderly victims (Miller et al. 1981; Ollendick and Hoffman 1982; Phifer and Norris 1989; Phifer et al. 1988; Shore et al. 1986). However, the majority of studies have not found that these consequences are more severe for the elderly. For example, in two studies that specifically addressed psychiatric symptomatology in older and younger disaster victims, no age differences were found. Ollendick and Hoffman found that both their older (mean age, 74; $n = 73$) and younger (mean age, 42; $n = 51$) groups reported increased symptoms of depression following a flood than they had during an evaluation before the flood, but that there were no differences between the groups in the degree of increase. Similarly, Miller et al. assessed specific symptoms in groups of older adults and younger adults 1 year following the 1976 Big Thompson flood in Colorado and found no significant differences between groups in the degree of loss sustained or in overall psychiatric symptomatology.

In a number of studies, fewer negative consequences were reported among elderly victims. For example, Bell (1978) found that younger (i.e., 18–59) victims of a tornado reported more physical and emotional indicators of stress than older victims. Likewise, Bolin and Klenow (1982–1983) found that reports of family disruption and nervousness were similar among younger and older victims during bad weather, but found lower scores on other measures of disaster-related symptomatology among the older victims (e.g., anxiety about future disasters). Gleser et al. (1981) reported more negative effects in their 25- to 54-year-old group compared with those above age 55 or below age 24 following the Buffalo Creek dam collapse, and Phifer (1990) found that subjects in the 55- to 64-year-old group reported more distress than those in the 65–74 or 75+ groups 18 months following a flood in Kentucky.

Explanations for a possible "protective" role of age often focus on the fact that different disasters may produce different types of stress in individuals of different age groups (Gibbs 1989). For example, Gleser et al. (1981) suggested that the middle-age adult subjects in their sample of survivors may have been most at risk for posttraumatic adjustment difficulties because younger adults had sufficient time to "start over" elsewhere whereas the older subjects may have had more limited ambitions. Findings of increased stress following disasters among younger adults who are in their childbearing years have also been reported in studies of residents of the Three Mile Island area (Bromet and Schulberg 1986; Cleary and Houts 1984), where there was a nuclear accident near Harrisburg, Pennsylvania, in March 1979.

Experience with a previous disaster may also contribute to a "protective" influence of age (Phifer and Norris 1989; Taylor and Frazer 1982). Phifer and Norris (1989) found that experience with a prior disaster promoted adaptation to a subsequent one. As Bell (1978) and Melick and Logue (1985–1986) suggested, healthy elderly persons may actually find more productive roles within their families and communities following disasters, which might, as a result, improve their overall adjustment. However, as Gibbs (1989) pointed out, this prior experience is only helpful if the previous trauma was dealt with successfully. For example, Hannsson et al. (1982) found that increased age and previous flood experience were associated with increased fear of future floods among residents of an Oklahoma flood plain. They speculated that among some individuals who were negatively affected by a previous disaster, the prospect of a subsequent disaster heightens their anxiety. Presumably, for others, successful "mastery" of a previous negative event might lead to increased confidence for the future. Other factors that might contribute to positive adjustment following trauma have been reviewed by Lyons (1991). These include the ability to reexperience a trauma with a "relatively high degree of voluntary control" (p. 98), the capacity to find meaning in some outcome of the trauma, and the availability of a social support system that is congruent with their needs.

Perhaps the best way of exploring the role that age plays in determining outcome following disaster is in the context of other variables. Studies of traumatic stress reactions consistently point to the importance of the type and severity of the trauma and preexisting variables when predicting outcome. For example, a study of residents of the St. Louis, Missouri, area who experienced flood and dioxin exposure in 1982 (Smith et al. 1986) found that victims of a flood reported a "full recovery" twice as often as those exposed to dioxin (whether or not they were also exposed to a flood). In addition, they found that although trauma exposure produced new PTSD symptoms regardless of prior exposure to trauma, increased depressive symptoms were noted only in those with a history of depression. Similarly, preexisting psychiatric, family, and behavioral problems were cited by Breslau et al. (1991) as risk factors for both the likelihood of experiencing trauma as well as for developing PTSD following it.

Among older adults, Bolin and Klenow (1988) found that socioeconomic status, marital status, availability of family and friends, and social support all correlated with emotional recovery for both elderly and nonelderly whites. These and other variables were, however, of differing importance within specific age and racial groups. The most comprehensive study of physical and psychological sequelae following natural disasters among the elderly to date is one in which 200 older residents (i.e., age 55 and older) of Kentucky were assessed prior to and four times following a flood of moderate severity in 1981 and 18 months following a severe flood in 1984 (Phifer 1990; Phifer and Norris 1989; Phifer et al. 1988). Both physical and psychological consequences were related to the severity of the flood (Phifer and Norris 1989); however, prior symptom level was the best overall predictor of eventual outcome. Regarding psychological consequences, three scales (State-Trait Anxiety, Center for Epidemiological Studies-Depression, General Well Being) were used to track emotional dysfunction following the floods.

In keeping with Smith et al. (1986), prior psychiatric symptom level was the strongest predictor of postflood symptom level, accounting for 30%–40% of the variance (Phifer 1990). The correlation between pre- and postflood physical status was even greater: 50%–70% of the variance in postdisaster physical status was accounted for by prior health status, whereas the severity of the flood accounted for only 2%–12% of the variance. With regard to age, Phifer reported that demographic variables (including age) accounted for only 3% of the variance in psychological symptoms following the severe flood in 1984. Furthermore, in this sample, it was the youngest of the three group samples (55–64, 65–74, 75+) that was at greatest risk.

To summarize, despite early reports of increased negative outcome and consistent findings of increased risk for physical harm among the elderly, the data of the past two decades do not support the hypothesis that older adults are at greater risk than younger adults for negative psychosocial outcome following exposure to natural disasters. The available data suggest that elderly persons cope as well, and at times better, than younger adults. These data suggest further that age contributes minimally to the prediction of psychosocial outcome and that variables such as preexisting physical and mental health, severity of trauma, and availability of specific resources are of greater predictive value. This is not to say that there are no differences in the way in which the elderly experience and respond to a traumatic experience. Based on differential life experiences and cohort factors, the elderly may have unique needs that should be taken into account by disaster relief workers. However, as of this writing, there is insufficient evidence to conclude that disaster causes more negative psychosocial consequences in older adults.

Environmental Relocation as a Traumatic Event

Although the literature of the past decade has failed to provide adequate or convincing evidence of an increased risk of anxiety, PTSD, or other postdisaster disorders among the elderly, there is clear evidence that the elderly are at risk for greater cognitive and physical decline than younger adults. One consequence of this decline for many elderly persons is the need to move to an environment that can provide them with assistance for their needs. Fields (1992) operationalized "reactive

environmental changes" (p. 519) as those that are "1) trig-
gered by life or environmental events (e.g., chronic illness,
functional decline, widowhood, condominium conversion),
2) designed to provide greater access to needed or anticipated
services, and 3) more common among the elderly than nonelderly" (p. 520), and cited relocation to nursing homes or
senior citizen apartments as examples.

When the elderly have control over these environmental
changes, when they have ample time and support to prepare
for them, and when these moves result in an improved congru-
ence between an individual's needs and the resources available
to them in their environment, most do reasonably well (Fields
1992). However, when these conditions are not met, some elderly persons do quite poorly. In fact, early reports of mortality
rates for elderly persons admitted or transferred to institutional settings were strikingly high (Carmago and Preston
1945; Whittier and Williams 1956). Despite methodological
weaknesses of these studies, numerous "transplantation
shock" studies followed and gave rise to one of the most heated
debates in the field of gerontology: that is, are the elderly at
greater risk for negative outcome (including mortality) following relocation or has the role of control and other factors in
determining outcome been exaggerated by methodological
problems and poor care in a few selected institutional settings
(Borup and Gallego 1981; Bourestom and Pastalan 1981;
Coffman 1983; Horowitz and Schulz 1983)?

The literature in this area is reviewed in detail elsewhere
(Coffman 1983; Fields 1992). Of relevance to the topic of this
chapter is whether adjustment difficulties following relocation
can be better understood from a PTSD perspective. The diagnosis of PTSD assumes a specific stressor. Typically, this stress-
or is a negative event over which the individual experiencing it
has little or no control. Although DSM-III-R (American Psychiatric Association 1987) enumerates the criteria necessary
for reaching a diagnosis, the phenomenology of PTSD is such
that a specific event produces lasting event-related effects
(e.g., reexperiences of or preoccupation with the trauma,

avoidant behavior, heightened arousal) as well as more generalized psychiatric distress or adjustment problems or both. It
seems quite plausible that forced relocation to a nursing home
might be experienced by some elderly persons as a traumatic
event. Early studies reported high mortality rates following
moves to an institution (Carmago and Preston 1945; Whittier
and Williams 1956), and more recent studies have documented the presence of depression in a significant proportion
of nursing home residents (Parmelee et al. 1989). However,
whether these individuals have specific symptoms of PTSD
has not been addressed. The fact that improvement in well-being has been reported among nursing home residents following
the initiation of programs designed to increase sense of control
over one's circumstances (Langer and Rodin 1976; Rodin et al.
1985; Schulz 1976) provides evidence that some symptoms
appearing after a relocation may be part of a treatable condition. Future attempts to conceptualize these symptoms from a
PTSD perspective may lead to initial studies of the prevalence
of PTSD symptomatology among nursing home residents as
well as the application of PTSD treatment strategies to this
population.

Summary

In this chapter, the issue of whether the elderly are at greater
risk for negative psychiatric and psychosocial consequences
following exposure to a traumatic event has been addressed.
Based on very limited epidemiological data, there is insufficient evidence to conclude that PTSD (or any other anxiety
disorder) is more common in the elderly. Similarly, based on
methodologically limited data, there is insufficient evidence to
conclude that community-dwelling, cognitively intact elderly
persons are at greater risk for negative psychosocial consequences following exposure to a natural disaster. These conclusions should not, however, steer clinicians and researchers
away from the topic of PTSD in the elderly. On the contrary,

the current review of this literature reveals the tremendous dearth of information in this area. Based on the data reviewed earlier, future studies may benefit clinicians who work with the elderly by assessing both the prevalence of the diagnosis PTSD as well as the prevalence of specific symptoms that may be related to trauma among older adults. Clinicians may also help their patients by including questions regarding previous experience of trauma as well as past and current symptoms of PTSD in their evaluation process. Finally, by considering experiences such as nursing home relocation from a PTSD perspective, new approaches to treating difficult problems unique to the elderly may arise.

References

Abrams R: Anxiety and personality disorders, in Comprehensive Review of Geriatric Psychiatry. Edited by Sadavoy J, Lazarus LW, Jarvik LF. Washington, DC, American Psychiatric Press, 1991, pp 369–386

American Psychiatric Association: Diagnostic and Statistical Manual of Mental Disorders, 3rd Edition. Washington, DC, American Psychiatric Association, 1980

American Psychiatric Association: Diagnostic and Statistical Manual of Mental Disorders, 3rd Edition, Revised. Washington, DC, American Psychiatric Association, 1987

Baum A, Gatchel RJ, Schaeffer MA: Emotional, behavioral, and physiological effects of chronic stress at Three Mile Island. J Consult Clin Psychol 51:565–572, 1983

Bell BD: Disaster impact and response: overcoming the thousand natural shocks. Gerontologist 18:531–539, 1978

Blazer D, George LK, Hughes D: The epidemiology of anxiety disorders: an age comparison, in Anxiety in the Elderly. Edited by Salzman C, Lebowitz BD. New York, Springer, 1991, pp 17–30

Bolin R: Response to natural disasters, in Health Response to Mass Emergencies: Theories and Practice. Edited by Lystand ML. New York, Brunner/Mazel, 1988, pp 22–51

Bolin R, Klenow DJ: Response of the elderly to disaster: an age stratified analysis. Int J Aging Hum Dev 16:283–296, 1982–1983

Bolin R, Klenow DJ: Older people in disaster: a comparison of black and white victims. Int J Aging Hum Dev 26:29–43, 1988

Borup JH, Gallego DT: Mortality as affected by interinstitutional relocation: update and assessment. Gerontologist 21:8–16, 1981

Bourestom N, Pastalan L: The effects of relocation on the elderly: a reply to Borup, Gallego and Hefferman. Gerontologist 2:4–7, 1981

Breslau N, Davis GL, Andreski P, et al: Traumatic events and posttraumatic stress disorder in an urban population of young adults. Arch Gen Psychiatry 48:216–222, 1991

Brickman AL, Eisdorfer C: Anxiety in the elderly, in Geriatric Psychiatry. Edited by Busse EW, Blazer DG. Washington, DC, American Psychiatric Press, 1989, pp 415–427

Bromet EJ, Schulberg HC: The Three Mile Island disaster: a search for high risk groups, in Disaster Stress Studies: New Methods and Findings. Edited by Shore JH. Washington, DC, American Psychiatric Press, 1986, pp 1–20

Busse EW, Blazer DG: Geriatric Psychiatry. Washington, DC, American Psychiatric Press, 1989

Carmago O, Preston GH: What happens to patients who are hospitalized for the first time when over sixty-five? Am J Psychiatry 102:168–173, 1945

Carter AO, Millson ME, Allen DE: Epidemiologic study of deaths and injuries due to tornadoes. Am J Epidemiology 130:1209–1218, 1989

Cleary PD, Houts PS: The psychological impact of Three Mile Island. Journal of Human Stress 10:28–34, 1984

Coffman TL: Toward an understanding of geriatric relocation. Gerontologist 23:453–459, 1983

Cohen ES, Poulshock SW: Societal response to mass relocation of the elderly. Gerontologist 17:262–268, 1977

Fields RB: Psychosocial response to environment change, in Handbook of Social Development: A Lifespan Perspective. Edited by Van Hasselt VB, Hersen M. New York, Plenum, 1992, pp 503–544

Frederick CJ: Effects of natural vs. human induced violence upon victims, in Evaluation and Change: Services for Survivors. Edited by Kivens L. Minneapolis, MN, Minneapolis Research Foundation, 1980, pp 71–75

Friedsam H: Reactions of older persons to disaster caused losses: an hypothesis of relative deprivation. Gerontologist 1:34–37, 1961

Friedsam HJ: Older persons in disaster, in Man and Society in Disaster. Edited by Baker GW, Chapman DW. New York, Basic Books, 1962, pp 151–182

Gaitz CM, Scott J: Age and the measurement of mental health. J Health Soc Behav 13:55–67, 1972

Gibbs MS: Factors in the victim that mediate between disaster and psychopathology: a review. Journal of Traumatic Stress 2:489–514, 1989

Gleser G, Green BL, Winget CN: Prolonged Psychological Effects of Disaster. New York, Academic Press, 1981

Green BL: Evaluating the effects of disasters. Psychological Assessment 3:538–546, 1991

Green BL, Lindy JD, Grace MC, et al: Buffalo Creek survivors in the second decade: stability of stress symptoms. Am J Orthopsychiatry 60:43–54, 1990

Hansson RO, Noulles D, Bellovich SJ: Knowledge, warning and stress: a study of comparative roles in an urban floodplain. Environment and Behavior 14:171–185, 1982

Helzer J, Robins LN, McEvoy L: Post-traumatic stress disorder in the general population. N Engl J Med 317:1630–1634, 1987

Horowitz MJ, Schulz R: The relocation controversy: criticism and commentary on five recent studies. Gerontologist 23:229–233, 1983

Huerta F, Horton R: Coping behavior of elderly flood victims. Gerontologist 18:541–546, 1978

Hutton J: The differential distribution of death in disaster: a test of theoretical propositions. Mass Emergencies 1:254–261, 1976

Jordan BK, Schlenger WE, Hough R, et al: Lifetime and current prevalence of specific psychiatric disorders among Vietnam veterans and controls. Arch Gen Psychiatry 48:207–215, 1991

Kilijanek TS, Drabek TE: Assessing long term impacts of a natural disaster: a focus on the elderly. Gerontologist 19:555–566, 1979

Langer EJ, Rodin J: The effects of choice and enhanced personal responsibility for the aged: a field experiment in an institutional setting. J Pers Soc Psychol 34:191–198, 1976

Leighton DC, Harding JS, Macklin DB, et al: The Character of Danger: Psychiatric Symptoms in Selected Communities, III. New York, Basic Books, 1963

Lifton RJ, Olson E: The human meaning of total disaster. Psychiatry 39:1–18, 1976

Lyons JA: Strategies for assessing the potential for positive adjustment following trauma. Journal of Traumatic Stress 4:93–111, 1991

Magni G, DeLeo D: Anxiety and depression in geriatric and adult medical inpatients: a comparison. Psychol Rep 55:607–612, 1984

McFarlane AC: Post-traumatic stress disorder. International Review of Psychiatry 3:203–313, 1991

Melick ME, Logue JN: The effect of disaster on health and well-being of older women. Int J Aging Hum Dev 21:27–38, 1985–1986

Miller JA, Turner JG, Kimball E: Big Thompson flood victims: one year later. Family Relations 30:111–116, 1981

Moore H, Friedsam H: Reported emotional stress following a disaster. Social Forces 38:135–139, 1959

Ollendick DG, Hoffman M Sr: Assessment of psychological reactions in disaster victims. Journal of Community Psychology 10:157–167, 1982

Parmelee PA, Katz I, Lawton MP: Depression among institutionalized aged: assessment and prevalence estimation. J Gerontol 44:M22–M29, 1989

Phifer JF: Psychological distress and somatic symptoms after natural disaster: differential vulnerability among older adults. Psychol Aging 5:412–420, 1990

Phifer JF, Norris FH: Psychological symptoms in older adults following natural disaster: nature, timing, duration, and course. J Gerontol 44:S207–S217, 1989

Phifer JF, Kaniasty KZ, Norris FH: The impact of natural disaster on the health of older adults: a multiwave prospective study. J Health Soc Behav 29:65–78, 1988

Regier DA, Boyd JH, Burke JD Jr, et al: One month prevalence of mental disorders in the United States. Arch Gen Psychiatry 45:977–986, 1988

Rodin J, Timko C, Harris S: The construct of control: biological and psychological correlates, in Annual Review of Gerontology and Geriatrics. Edited by Lawton MP, Madox GL. New York, Springer, 1985, pp 3–55

Rosen J, Fields RB, Hand AM, et al: Concurrent posttraumatic stress disorder in psychogeriatric patients. J Geriatr Psychiatry Neurol 2:65–69, 1989

Sadavoy J, Lazarus LW, Jarvik LF: Comprehensive Review of Geriatric Psychiatry. Washington, DC, American Psychiatric Press, 1991

Salzman C, Lebowitz BD: Anxiety in the Elderly. New York, Springer, 1991

Schulz R: Effects of control and predictability on the physical and psychological well-being of the institutionalized aged. J Pers Soc Psychol 33:563–573, 1976

Shamoian CA: What is anxiety in the elderly?, in Anxiety in the Elderly. Edited by Salzman L, Lebowitz BD. New York, Springer, 1991, pp 1–15

Shore JH, Tatum E, Vollmer W: Psychiatric reactions to disaster: the Mt. St. Helens experience. Am J Psychiatry 143: 590–595, 1986

Shore JH, Vollmer WM, Tatum EL: Community patterns of post traumatic stress disorders. J Nerv Ment Dis 177:681–685, 1989

Sierles FS, Chen JJ, MacFarland RE, et al: Posttraumatic stress disorder and concurrent psychiatric illness: a preliminary report. Am J Psychiatry 140:1177–1179, 1983

Smith EM, Robins LN, Pryzbeck TR, et al: Psychosocial consequences of a disaster, in Disaster Stress Studies: New Methods and Findings. Edited by Shore JH. Washington, DC, American Psychiatric Press, 1986, pp 50–76

Smith EM, North CS, Price PC: Response to technological accidents, in Mental Health Response to Mass Emergencies: Theories and Practice. Edited by Lystad ML. New York, Brunner/Mazel, 1988, pp 52–95

Taylor AJW, Frazer AG: The stress of past-disaster body handling and victim identification work. Journal of Human Stress 8:4–12, 1982

Warheit GJ, Bell RA, Schwab JJ, et al: An epidemiologic assessment of mental health problems in the southeastern United States, in Community Surveys of Psychiatric Disorders. Edited by Weissman MM, Myers JK, Ross CE. New Brunswick, NJ, Rutgers University Press, 1986, pp 191–208

Whittier JR, Williams D: The coincidence and constancy of mortality figures for aged psychotic patients admitted to state hospitals. J Nerv Ment Dis 124:618–620, 1956

Zubin J, Spring B: Vulnerability: a new view of schizophrenia. J Abnorm Psychol 86:103–126, 1977

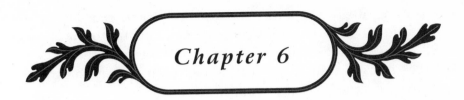

Chapter 6

Age-Related Reactions to the Buffalo Creek Dam Collapse

Effects in the Second Decade

Bonnie L. Green, Ph.D.,
Goldine C. Gleser, Ph.D.,
Jacob D. Lindy, M.D.,
Mary C. Grace, M.Ed., M.S., and
Anthony Leonard, B.A.

Evidence has been accumulating over the past decade that, contrary to intuition and anecdotal reports (e.g., Cohen and Ahearn 1980), elderly victims of disasters may not be at particularly high risk for developing emotional problems following disaster. As a matter of fact, it presently seems as if they may have a better prognosis than their younger counterparts. However, the findings have not been conclusive, and rarely have groups of various ages,

The work reported in this chapter was supported by National Institute of Mental Health Grants R01 MH26321 (to Dr. Gleser) and R01 MH40401 (to Dr. Green).

including subgroups of older adults, been compared. The present study included a wide age range of adults up to the age of 87 who could be compared for their responses to the Buffalo Creek disaster using data from a longitudinal study to explore changes over a 12-year period.

The Buffalo Creek dam collapse happened in the Buffalo Creek Valley, West Virginia, on a cold Saturday morning in February of 1972. It had been raining for several days, and rumors abounded about the possible breaking of the slag dam, but residents had been assured by officials that they were not in danger. However, at about 8 A.M., on the 26th, the dam gave way, inundating the narrow valley below with thousands of gallons of water and black sludge from the dam. Descriptions of the event suggest that it resembled a huge tidal wave, careening from one side of the valley to the other until it finally subsided and emptied into the Guyandotte River (Erikson 1976). When the flood waters had receded, 125 people had died, and thousands were left homeless.

Residents banded together to sue the coal company in a landmark legal case that has become a common part of law school curricula (Stern 1976). The sample reported on here represents subsamples of litigants and nonlitigants from the original legal action, some of whom were studied by our research team in 1974 (Gleser et al. 1981) and followed up 14 years after the event in 1986 (Green et al. 1990a, 1990b).

A few studies of disasters have shown higher risk for emotional problems in "older" subjects. For example, Leopold and Dillon (1963) found that, of survivors in a marine collision, those over the age of 35 were much more likely to get worse over time than those under age 35, comparing the initial response to the response at 4 years. Hansson et al. (1982) found older flood victims to be more psychologically distressed than younger victims, and Price (1978) found victims in the 36–74 age range to be the most distressed. He suggested that this was because they were more likely to be property owners. The age ranges in these studies were quite broad, however, and subjects being defined as "older" were sometimes quite young. Kilijanek and Drabek (1979) studied tornado victims 3 years following a tornado in Kansas, dividing subjects into age groups of 39 or less, 40–59, and 60 or older. The elderly in this sample showed a "pattern of neglect"; that is, they received fewer services than the other groups. Although the subjects over 60 reported fewer self-rated physical symptoms than the sample of nonvictims, they had more health complaints than their younger counterparts. With regard to "anomia" (alienation), the older subjects were more alienated than their younger counterparts, but no more alienated than nonvictims. Thus, there was no evidence that their greater alienation and physical complaints resulted from the trauma of the disaster.

Other studies found differences that went in the opposite direction. For example, Taylor and Frazer (1982) studied body handlers after an airline crash and found that both immediately and at 20 months, older subjects were less distressed than younger subjects. Likewise, Green et al. (1985), studying survivors of a supper club fire, found that older subjects were less at risk for developing psychological symptoms at 1 and 2 years. This was particularly true of self-rated symptom distress (and particularly hostility symptoms) and for interviewer ratings of substance abuse.

A number of studies have compared older (usually 60 years and up) to younger subjects, specifically investigating the reactions of elderly adults. Generally, the findings support the notion that these individuals do well relative to their younger cohorts. Bell (1978) found that 18–30 weeks following a tornado, survivors over the age of 60 were less stressed and anxious than those under 60. Six months following the Teton Dam collapse, Huerta and Horton (1978) found no differences in grieving over losses between survivors 65 and older and those younger than 65, but the older subjects felt that they were more recovered from the flood effects. Samples of older (60 and up) survivors of two tornadoes studied by Bolin and Klenow (1982–1983) showed fewer psychological symptoms (e.g., nervousness, bad dreams) than younger (below 60) subjects. This occurred despite the fact that this group felt more loss (although they did not objectively suffer more material losses) and were in fact more likely to have been injured or suffered a tornado-related death in their household or both. Perhaps it is for these latter objective reasons that the older group did not feel more recovered, even though they reported significantly fewer symptoms than the younger subjects at 1 year after the tornado. Ollendick and Hoffmann (1982) found no differences between their survivors of a flash flood over the age of 60 compared with younger subjects on a symptom checklist.

A few studies have tried to make finer distinctions with regard to age in examining samples of disaster survivors to ascertain whether any particular age group is more at risk, rather than looking simply at a linear relationship or comparing elderly survivors to all others. Norris et al. (1994) studied, prospectively, a group of older adults exposed to a series of floods in eastern Kentucky. Subjects were 55 years or older at the time that the study was initiated (average, 67 years). Examining the subjects by age group, they found that the subjects ages 55–64 were most affected by the disasters, as indicated by scores on a depression scale. Adults age 65–74 were affected very little, whereas their oldest group (75+) was affected to an intermediate degree. This suggests that relationships with age may not be linear and that there may be particular groups of adults who are more at risk for various reasons.

Logue et al. (1981) also found that their subjects ages 55–64 had the most mental health problems following exposure to Hurricane Agnes in 1972, based on a mail survey using the Zung, the Langner, and the SCL-90 scales administered about 5 years following the disaster.

In our initial study 2 years after the Buffalo Creek dam collapse, we examined the findings by age group to determine whether any of the age groups were particularly at risk for psychological sequelae of the collapse. Subjects were divided into four age groups: 16–24, 25–39, 40–54, and 55 and older at time of the flood. Regardless of the symptoms studied, the two middle-age groups were doing the worst. The 40–54 age group showed the most anxiety symptoms, and the 25–39 age group showed the most belligerence symptoms, according to ratings made by the research team (Gleser et al. 1981). Men and women varied with regard to which age group was most at risk for depression and overall severity. In each case, the curvilinear trend was significant. Our 14 year follow-up study allows us to examine a subgroup of this original sample to see whether recovery from the disaster differed by age group.

Methods

The original data were collected in the context of a lawsuit against the coal company that built the collapsed slag dam. Residents were interviewed by mental health professionals from both sides of the lawsuit between 18 and 26 months after the flood. Both sets of reports were used to rate 1974 psychopathology (Gleser et al. 1981). The lawsuit was settled out of court in the summer of 1974. In 1986, we returned to interview many of the original 381 adults originally seen.

Subjects

Of the original 381 adult plaintiffs, 120 were located and completed a valid interview. Because 52 of the original plaintiffs had died, this figure represented 39% of living survivors. Of those living survivors not interviewed, 33% were known to have moved out of state; 36% refused; and 32% could not be accounted for, were never contacted, or could not be scheduled for an interview (Green and Grace 1988). Based on 1974 reports, survivors who participated in the follow-up had suffered significantly less personal loss through death during the flood than had those who refused to participate. However, there were no differences between participants and refusers in the level of 1974 clinically rated or self-reported psychopathology (Green and Grace 1988).

Comparison Samples

In 1986, in addition to the original subjects, a sample of
78 flood survivors was recruited who had not participated in
the lawsuit. The litigants and nonlitigants were similar on
nearly all dimensions including demographic characteristics,
degree of exposure to life threat and loss due to the dam collapse, and their levels of self-reported and rated functioning
(Green et al. 1990a). Also, with one exception, rates of disorder did not vary significantly between the two groups. The
group that sued had slightly higher rates of generalized anxiety disorder than did the group that did not sue (Green et al.
1990a).

Finally, a group of culturally similar residents from Boone,
Raleigh, and Kanawha counties in West Virginia were
recruited, with help from the Family and Community Health
Department at Marshall University, as a comparison group.
These subjects showed lower rates of anxiety, depression, and
hostility symptoms and diagnoses than the two exposed samples (Green et al. 1990a).

Measures

The instruments described in this report are those on which
we had comparable data in 1974 and 1986 and entailed only
a portion of the entire protocol from 1986.

Clinical ratings.   In 1974, the diagnostic interviews were
rated on the Psychiatric Evaluation Form (PEF) (Endicott and
Spitzer 1972; Spitzer et al. 1968). The PEF consists of 19 rating scales of different clinical symptoms (e.g., anxiety, depression, suicidal thoughts, grandiosity) as well as a rating of
overall severity. Each rating is made on a scale from 1 to 6
(none to extreme impairment). A factor analysis from an earlier outpatient study had shown the symptoms to cluster into
three areas. These clusters, with minor changes, were retained

for the 1974 Buffalo Creek study. The clusters were depression (from the scales of depression, suicide/self-mutilation, social isolation, daily routine impairment, and retardation/lack of emotion), anxiety (from agitation-excitement, anxiety, and somatic concerns), and belligerence (from suspicion/persecution, belligerence, and antisocial attitudes and acts). Overall severity and alcohol abuse were used separately.

Interrater generalizability (rho-squared) was estimated to range between .60 (for overall severity) and .90 depending on the scale, using one rater, randomly assigned, for each interview (Cronbach et al. 1972).

Correlations between ratings on the two reports (done in different settings, at different times, and for different sides of the lawsuit) ranged from .28 to .56 for the summary scores (Gleser et al. 1981), indicating valid individual differences among the litigants. Because the average of the two scores would reduce error stemming from the differences in the style and perspectives of the two reports, this was seen as the best information regarding the individual's psychopathology. We therefore combined the scores from the two sides of the suit.

In 1986, the PEF ratings were made following a structured psychiatric interview for diagnosis. The rating scales were combined into the same cluster scores used in the prior study. Generalizability for the summary scores ranged from .75 to .90 and for overall severity was .66.

Symptom self-report.   The 47-item checklist used in 1974 was based on an earlier version of the SCL-90. At that time, average symptom intensity was used as the self-report measure of subjective distress. Although the research plan called for each person to fill out the SCL, this was not always done; thus, the number of SCL scores available to examine change is lower than that for the clinical ratings. In 1986, the SCL-90R (Derogatis 1983) was used as the self-report symptom index. A few items missing from that index that were rated in 1974 were added so that change on the original 47 items could be assessed. Subscales based on the 47-item checklist included scales for somatic symptoms, anxiety, depression, hostility, obsessive-compulsive symptoms, and an overall severity score.

Diagnosis. The Structured Clinical Interview for DSM-III (SCID) (Spitzer and Williams 1986) is a diagnostic interview designed to be used by individuals with clinical training. It covers all major Axis I diagnoses and in 1986 had already been modified to address most of the DSM-III-R criteria (American Psychiatric Association 1987). A posttraumatic stress disorder (PTSD) section was then in development by the authors of the instrument, and this version was somewhat modified by our research team after several trials because the original did not distinguish well enough between intrusive images and voluntary recollections. Our modified version, with the additional DSM-III-R symptoms, was subsequently adopted in the general interview schedule and was used in the validation portion of a national study of Vietnam veterans (Kulka et al. 1990).

   In 1974, there was no diagnosis of PTSD in the psychiatric nosology. However, because the diagnosticians on both sides of the lawsuit were aware of the diagnoses of traumatic neurosis and transient stress reactions, symptoms of these disorders, if present, were routinely documented in the reports. For our 1986 study, the earlier reports were examined, and diagnoses of PTSD were assigned. However, a structured interview for diagnosis was not used in 1974, and not all symptoms in the current criteria were covered, especially not those that have been added most recently to the criteria (e.g., sense of foreshortened future). Thus, a more liberal criterion had to be developed for the retrospective diagnosis. To receive a PTSD diagnosis from the 1974 reports, the subject had to evidence one intrusion symptom from DSM-III (American Psychiatric Association 1980) or DSM-III-R, two denial symptoms (numbing or avoidance), and one additional physiological arousal symptom. Interrater reliability for these retrospective diagnoses was .68 (kappa). Records were scored by one person, and questionable protocols were reviewed by at least two members of the research team. In addition to psychopathology, ratings of aspects of each subject's stressor experience during the dam collapse were made from information in the 1974 reports and additional questions in the 1986 interview.

Interviewers

Interviewers were seven women and four men. Six were graduate students in clinical psychology. Two graduate students in other fields and three bachelor's- or master's-level individuals with prior interviewing experience also served as interviewers. Extensive interviewer training was conducted, including sensitization to the culture and the general trauma experience of the survivors, training in administration and scoring of the SCID, and practice interviews among the interviewers and with outpatient psychiatric patients.

Procedure

Four data collection trips were made to the Buffalo Creek area between February and July of 1986. Attempts were made to follow individuals who still lived within a 60-mile radius of the valley. Subjects gave their informed consent before being interviewed, and interviews lasted from 90 minutes to 3 hours, including all instruments. Subjects were provided referral information about the local mental health center when appropriate.

Results

Longitudinal Analyses

Subjects were divided into approximately equal age groups depending on their age at the time of the flood: 16–23 (30–37 at follow-up in 1986), 24–38 (38–52 in 1986), 39–49 (53–63 in 1986), and 50 or older (64 or older in 1986). These groups correspond roughly to the age groups used for the 1974 data (Gleser et al. 1981), although some of the older subjects had died, reducing this age pool somewhat.

Current demographic characteristics of the four groups can be seen in Table 6–1. The groups were similar in terms of gender proportion of each group, marital status, extent of flood-related life threat, and number of moves in the 2 years following the flood. They differed with regard to education; the older groups were less educated. Also, older subjects tended to be living alone more often ($P < .06$) and to have reported slightly lower loss (bereavement) of friends and loved ones in the flood. These latter variables were used as covariates in some of the analyses.

In our 1974 study (Gleser et al. 1981), men and women showed different degrees of impairment that were, generally speaking, sex-role linked. Women showed higher anxiety and depression (and overall symptomatology), and men showed higher belligerence and alcohol-related problems. In 1986, women's scores had decreased more than those of men (Green

Table 6–1. Demographic characteristics of 120 Buffalo Creek survivors by age group at time of disaster

| | Age group | | | |
| | 16–23 | 24–38 | 39–49 | 53–63 |
Characteristics	(N = 27)	(N = 28)	(N = 33)	(N = 32)
Female (%)	67	54	67	59
Married (%)	82	75	73	66
Living alone (%)[*]	7	0	21	16
Education (N years)[**]	11.7	10.0	7.4	8.3
Life threat in disaster (1–5)	3.0	3.1	3.4	2.9
Loss in disaster (0–4)[*]	2.1	2.0	1.9	1.5
Moves after disaster (N)	3.0	3.0	2.5	2.5

[*]$P < .07$ for age differences by analysis of variance.
[**]$P < .01$ by analysis of variance.

et al. 1990b), although both groups showed significant decreases in rated and reported symptoms, and the two groups looked quite similar, implying some gender-linked differences in recovery. We therefore were interested in examining gender along with age when investigating recovery. In 1986, women continued to have somewhat higher PTSD rates than men (31% compared with 23%).

Analyses were run with and without the covariates (extent of flood-related bereavement, living arrangement [alone or with others], and level of education) because these variables tended to differ by group. Results of the analyses were virtually identical; therefore statistics are presented for those analyses controlling for the variables mentioned. All means presented are original raw means.

PEF.   Multivariate analyses of covariance were conducted for the three summary PEF scores separately, for overall severity, and for the PTSD diagnosis, with gender and age group as between-subject factors and time (1974, 1986) as the within-subject factor.

Table 6–2 shows the results of these analyses on the 117 subjects with complete PEF data and covariate data at the two time points. Somewhat fewer cases were available for analysis of the PTSD variable. For all variables, the change from 1974 to 1986 was significant ($P < .001$).

Results within the PEF were quite consistent, with the exception of belligerence. There were overall differences between men and women with regard to anxiety, depression, and overall severity. This difference held for the PTSD diagnosis as well. In all cases, the women showed higher means (higher symptom ratings) than the men. Although, as mentioned earlier, this difference was less in 1986 than in 1974, the gender-by-time interactions were not significant. None of these variables showed age group effects or age-group-by-time interactions.

The PEF variables (except belligerence) did show a three-way interaction of gender and age group with time (*F*s ranging

Table 6–2. Multivariate analysis of covariance results on Psychiatric Evaluation Form ratings and Posttraumatic stress disorder (PTSD) diagnosis by four age groups, gender, and occasion ($N = 117$)

	Psychiatric Evaluation Form				PTSD ($N = 108$)
	Anxiety	Depression	Belligerence	Overall severity	
Between subjects					
Age group	NS	NS	NS	NS	NS
Gender	$P < .01$	$P < .05$	NS	$P < .10$	$P < .05$
Age group × gender	NS	NS	NS	NS	NS
Within subjects					
Age group × time	NS	NS	NS	NS	NS
Gender × time	NS	NS	NS	NS	NS
Age × gender × time	$P < .05$	$P < .01$	NS	$P < .01$	NS

Note. NS = not significant.

from 3.05 to 8.09, df = 3/109, Ps ranging from < .05 to < .001). The interaction was quite similar across measures and is graphed in Figure 6–1 for the overall severity measure. For three of the age groups, the recovery curves were quite similar, although women's scores in the youngest and oldest group were slightly higher than the men's. However, for those survivors between the ages of 24 and 38 at the time of the flood (38–52 at follow-up), men showed a weaker recovery than women. Women's scores started higher and ended up lower than those of the men. For anxiety, women's mean scores for the second age group went from 2.8 to 1.4, and men's scores went from 2.1 to 1.6. Depression scores went from 2.3 to 1.3 for women and from 1.7 to 1.6 for men.

SCL.   Initial (1974) symptom checklist scores were available only for 73 of the 120 subjects. Therefore, adjacent age groups

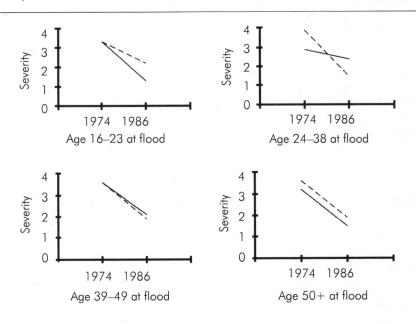

Figure 6–1.   Psychiatric Evaluation Form overall severity three-way interaction. Solid lines indicate men; broken lines indicate women.

Table 6–3. Multivariate analyses of covariance results on Symptom Checklist reports by two age groups, gender, and occasion ($N = 73$)

	Somatic	Anxiety	Hostility	Obsessive-compulsive	Depression	Total
Between subjects						
Age group	NS	NS	NS	NS	NS	NS
Gender	NS	NS	NS	NS	$P < .05$	NS
Age group × gender	NS	NS	NS	NS	NS	NS
Within subjects						
Age group × time	NS	NS	NS	$P < .10$	NS	NS
Gender × time	NS	$P < .05$	NS	$P < .05$	$P < .10$	$P < .10$
Age × gender × time	NS	NS	NS	NS	NS	NS

Note.   NS = not significant.

were collapsed to form two groups (16–38 and 39–50+). Table 6–3 shows the results of these analyses. In general, they are much weaker than those for the PEF, perhaps due to the lower Ns and also the collapsing of adjacent groups. Only one gender difference emerged: women reported more depression symptoms than men (women, 2.02–.90; men, 1.5–.83). On obsessive-compulsive symptoms, the older group had somewhat elevated symptoms relative to the younger group in 1974, but the groups were similar in 1986; however, this was a marginal finding. The gender-by-time findings for the anxiety symptoms reflect the fact that women started higher than men in 1974 and made a more dramatic decrease in symptoms (equal to or below that of men) in 1986.

Cross-Sectional Analyses

We decided to examine differences in a cross-sectional manner as well to see whether final status differed by age group. For these analyses, our N was larger because we could include all of the follow-up subjects as well as the newly recruited survivors who had not participated in the original lawsuit. Age groups were able to be somewhat more differentiated for this analysis: 16–21 at time of flood (30–35 at time of follow-up), 22–31, 32–41, 42–51, 52–61, and 62–73 (76–87 at time of follow-up). These groups differed on slightly different demographics than the earlier groups (education, living arrangement, number of moves following the disaster), which were controlled in the analyses. Covariance analyses were performed on the PEF (1986), the SCL-90 (1986), and the PTSD diagnosis.

Table 6–4 shows the results of these analyses, presenting three subscales of the SCL-90 along with the Global Severity Index, the overall severity rating from the PEF, and the current diagnosis of PTSD. It can be seen that, across the board, the group with the highest levels of problems, either rated or reported, were the adults in the 22–31 (at time of disaster)

Table 6–4. Mean symptoms and ratings by age group in adult survivors of Buffalo Creek (cross-sectional sample, $N = 179$)

Age group (at time of flood)	SCL-90				Global Severity Index*	Psychiatric Evaluation Form overall severity*	Diagnosis of posttraumatic stress disorder (%)
	N	Depression**	Anxiety*	Hostility**			
16–21	34	.89	.89	.68	.76	1.74	23
22–31	33	1.33	1.06	1.00	1.07	2.12	33
32–41	38	.87	.75	.50	.76	1.97	24
42–51	36	.85	.71	.44	.74	1.65	21
52–61	21	.65	.69	.27	.60	1.70	24
62–73	17	.58	.31	.18	.47	1.72	28

Note.   *$P < .05$, **$P < .01$ for age differences, by analysis of covariance, controlling for living arrangement, number of moves following the dam collapse (disruption), and level of education. Means in the table are uncorrected for the covariates.

group. The youngest age group, and those survivors between the ages of 32 and 41, showed similar levels of distress/functioning. The oldest age groups looked the best, with the eldest group (62 and older at flood, 76–87 at the time of the interview) showing the fewest problems. Two other SCL-90 scales also showed significant differences by age: paranoid ideation and interpersonal sensitivity. These scales showed similar trends to those in the table. The only exception was that for paranoid ideation; the eldest group showed somewhat elevated scores relative to the 52–61 age group. They were still lower than the three youngest groups. For interviewer-rated pathology on the PEF, not very many differences emerged. Overall severity, as noted in the table, showed significant age differences, but ratings of anxiety and depression did not. On alcohol abuse, differences were significant (P < .03), with the only group showing elevated drinking being those ages 22–31 at the time of the flood (36–45 in 1986). Memory impairment also differed, with the third age group (now 46–55) and the fifth age group (now 66–75) being rated as most memory impaired.

No differences were found between the groups on percentage of subjects meeting current criteria for a PTSD diagnosis. The diagnosis of alcohol abuse did differ by age group (P < .05), with the second age group, as in the other analyses, showing the highest rate (12% compared with 0–4% in the other groups). No other diagnostic differences were noted.

Questions about attempts to cope with the distress of the dam collapse revealed few differences. One difference that did emerge after controlling for the demographic and stress factors was the use of religion as a coping strategy (P < .01). Only 3%–4% of the three youngest groups selected this as their primary coping strategy, whereas 12% of the fourth age group and 18% of the fifth age group chose it. Finally, 43% of the oldest age group reported this as their primary coping strategy. The only other strategy that showed differences by age was that of helping others, where the group presently ages 56–65 reported the most use of this strategy (P < .02).

Questions about use of leisure or social time indicated that there was a linear trend with regard to going to church. Older subjects were much more likely than younger subjects to go to church ($P < .01$). Younger subjects were more likely to spend their time in active sporting activities or shopping and visiting others.

Discussion

The overall mental health of the Buffalo Creek survivors should be briefly reviewed so that the findings may be put in context. As noted, the group as a whole was functioning more poorly than a group of culturally similar subjects not exposed to a disaster (Green et al. 1990a). Of the Buffalo Creek survivors, 63% met lifetime criteria for disaster-related PTSD, and, at the time of the follow-up, 23% met current criteria. In addition, 21% of the sample met current criteria for major depression, 18% for generalized anxiety disorder, and 15% for simple phobia. The overall level of severity for those subjects meeting criteria for PTSD had declined between 1974 and 1986 (Green et al. 1990b). However, the group as a whole still scored higher than the general population sample on which the measure was normed on the SCL-90 Global Severity Index (Buffalo Creek, .81; comparison, .30). Thus, the sample on which we report continues to show notable psychological sequelae related to disaster status.

With regard to status in 1986, there were fairly clear-cut differences by age. The two oldest groups consistently showed the fewest effects. The group that showed the most impairment was the group ages 36–45 (22–31 at flood). These findings are similar to those in the original study: the middle-age group(s) showing the most impairment and the oldest group(s) the least.

By self-report, although not by interviewer rating, the very oldest age group (76–87) was doing even better than the next to oldest group (66–75), particularly with regard to anxiety symptoms. These findings in general are quite compatible with those of Norris et al. (1994), where subjects exposed to a Kentucky flood in the 55–64 age group (the youngest age group examined by these authors) had the most difficulty coping with losses in the floods as measured by symptoms of depression. In their study, the oldest adults (75+) were intermediate in their coping and those ages 65–74 did the best. In our study, the latter two groups were reversed. However, in both cases, the oldest groups (65+) were functioning relatively better than the younger group. In our study, the individuals in the 36–45 (22–31 at flood) age group were particularly at risk for problems.

Although the groups differed with regard to outcome (i.e., status in 1986), the differences in recovery by age were not impressive. No overall differences by age group emerged in patterns of recovery. On the other hand, gender emerged as a salient factor in recovery, primarily because women showed more anxiety and depression symptoms to begin with than men and thus made a more dramatic recovery. This gender difference was particularly notable in the age group that was between 24 and 38 at the time of the flood. From 1974 to 1986, women went from being rated as quite depressed and anxious to much lower levels. The curve for this age group was a bit steeper than for subjects (including women) in any of the other age groups. Men in this age group, on the other hand, essentially remained the same, whereas men in the other age groups improved. It is unfortunate that the Ns were so small for the symptom checklist data because combining the age groups may have obscured differences attributable to this one age group.

In trying to put together the longitudinal findings with the cross-sectional findings, one would need to focus on the group of younger middle-age adults as being particularly at risk. In terms of the 2-year data, the 25–39 age group had the highest belligerence symptoms, and the 40–54 age group showed the most anxiety. Women 25–39 were at very high risk for depression; depression for men was highest in the 40–54 age group.

Looking at status in 1986, those individuals 22–31 at the time of the disaster were having the most trouble, and all subjects under 52 were doing worse than the older groups. Although the longitudinal findings did not identify age-group-by-time effects, the men in the 24–38 age group at the time of the flood were the only ones who did not show a clear-cut recovery on the measures we used. Although shifting cutoffs for age groups is somewhat confusing, it is clear that the highest risk group includes those individuals in their 20s and 30s at the time of the disaster and that the older individuals (over 50) were not at particular risk.

In attempting to discuss possible reasons for these differences, it is difficult to know whether to concentrate on why older persons do better or why younger persons do worse. A number of potential explanations have been offered for differences in past disaster studies (see the beginning of this chapter), including differences in stressors during the disaster. However, in the present study, the differences between age groups in the amount of life threat or loss suffered and disruption (number of moves after the flood) was controlled statistically. Thus, differences in stressors are not a possible explanation for age differences in the present study.

Although it is possible that the age differences found in our and others' studies are specific to disaster adaptation, they more likely reflect differences among age groups in general. Comparison of this sample with a nonexposed comparison group showed that although absolute levels of symptoms varied by disaster status, age trends differed very little between the two groups (i.e., older subjects from the nonexposed group were doing better as well). Epidemiologic Catchment Area studies (Myers et al. 1984) likewise showed clear-cut differences by age in the general population with regard to psychiatric disorders. Men and women over age 45 showed lower rates of nearly all psychiatric disorders than those younger than 45. Except for cognitive impairment, the age group 65 years and above showed still lower rates of disorder than those 45–64.

Older adults may be at lower risk in general and in their response to stressors for a variety of reasons. Norris et al. (1994) discussed the possibility that older subjects have probably lived through crises in the past and that these experiences may have increased their resistance to subsequent stress because they have had the experience of coping successfully. In fact, they were able to demonstrate this finding in their data, where they found that more experienced older adults (i.e., those who had experienced some other traumatic event in their past) showed fewer effects from the flood than those with less experience. Our present study did examine an overall index of life stress experiences and found that these did not differ by age group. However, the data collected in this area were not as detailed as those collected by Norris et al., so their inferences regarding prior experience need to be given continued consideration.

In our study, we did find some differences between subjects in the various age groups that may help additionally to explain the better adaptation of older individuals. Specifically, the subjects in our two older age groups reported much higher rates than other age groups of turning to religion to cope with their distress about the disaster. Similarly, they were more likely to spend their leisure time attending church than the younger subjects. This drawing on religious beliefs for coping would be consistent with a more stoical or accepting attitude about the events surrounding the disaster and perhaps seeing the events that happened as "God's will" or as containing some lesson that needed to be learned. This may have had a particular calming effect and resulted in fewer attempts to blame responsible parties or causes in the external environment. There is also some suggestion that there may have been more positive effects of the flood for the elderly population. We asked an open-ended question about whether subjects saw any positive effect that came out of the disaster for them or for the community. Controlling for the variables noted in Table 6–4, the oldest group of subjects reported that they had benefited by having a more improved home or more money after the flood than before. A third of subjects in the oldest age group reported this aspect, whereas less than 10% of the other five age groups responded in this manner ($P < .05$). The eldest group, based on its low education and longevity in the community, may have had less adequate housing prior to the flood and may have benefited more by the rebuilding than the other groups.

The middle-age group, by contrast, may have had more of a burden placed on its members to care for others. This group (currently 36–45) was likely to have children in the home with them and, in this Appalachian community where families tend to live close to each other, may have had parents living in the home as well. Thus, the burden of responsibility was likely to be quite high for this group in particular. Further, the younger group, many of whom were coal miners, may have continued to have to work for the company that they believed caused the dam collapse that devastated their community. Older residents had probably retired at this point, undoubtedly reducing any conflict that potentially existed for individuals in this employment situation.

In conclusion, elderly disaster survivors appear to be at relatively low risk for developing long-term psychological problems following these events. Their coping strategies, and perhaps their cumulative past experience, seem to allow them to take changes brought on by the disaster events relatively in stride. Additionally, because they may have reduced burdens in terms of caring for others at this time, they may have fewer worries and more time to devote to dealing with the meaning and the resolution of the event. As always, those who have the most stressful experiences (e.g., loss or life threat, prolonged exposure) would be at higher risk than those not so exposed (Green et al. 1990b) and should be targeted for intervention on that basis. There is currently very little evidence, however, to support targeting older survivors based solely on their age. As a matter of fact, the findings indicate that these individuals may have a great deal to offer their younger family and friends in terms of a positive attitude and calming effect, and this resource should be considered and tapped.

References

American Psychiatric Association: Diagnostic and Statistical Manual of Mental Disorders, 3rd Edition. Washington, DC, American Psychiatric Association, 1980

American Psychiatric Association: Diagnostic and Statistical Manual of Mental Disorders, 3rd Edition, Revised. Washington, DC, American Psychiatric Association, 1987

Bell BD: Disaster impact and response: overcoming the thousand natural shocks. Gerontologist 18:531–540, 1978

Bolin R, Klenow DJ: Response of the elderly to disaster: an age-stratified analysis. Int J Aging Hum Dev 16:283–296, 1982–1983

Cohen RE, Ahearn FL Jr: Handbook for Mental Health Care of Disaster Victims. Baltimore, MD, Johns Hopkins University Press, 1980

Cronbach LJ, Gleser GC, Nanda H, et al: The Dependability of Behavioral Measurements: Theory of Generalizability for Scores and Profiles. New York, Wiley, 1972

Derogatis LR: SCL-90R Version: Manual I. Baltimore, MD, Johns Hopkins University, 1983

Endicott J, Spitzer R: What! another rating scale? the Psychiatric Evaluation Form. J Nerv Ment Dis 154:88–104, 1972

Erikson KT: Everything in Its Path. New York, Simon & Schuster, 1976

Gleser GC, Green BL, Winget C: Prolonged Psychosocial Effects of Disaster: A Study of Buffalo Creek. New York, Academic Press, 1981

Green BL, Grace MC: Conceptual issues in research with survivors and illustrations from a follow-up study, in Human Adaptation to Extreme Stress: From the Holocaust to Vietnam. Edited by Wilson JP, Harel Z, Kahana B. New York, Plenum, 1988, pp 105–124

Green BL, Grace MC, Gleser GC: Identifying survivors at risk: long-term impairment following the Beverly Hills Supper Club fire. J Consult Clin Psychol 53:672–678, 1985

Green BL, Grace MC, Lindy JD, et al: Buffalo Creek survivors in the second decade: comparison with unexposed and non-litigant groups. Journal of Applied Social Psychology 20:1033–1050, 1990a

Green BL, Lindy JD, Grace MC, et al: Buffalo Creek survivors in the second decade: stability of stress symptoms. Am J Orthopsychiatry 61:43–54, 1990b

Hansson RO, Noulles D, Bellovich SJ: Knowledge, warning and stress: a study of comparative roles in an urban flood-plain. Environment and Behavior 14:171–185, 1982

Huerta F, Horton R: Coping behavior of elderly flood victims. Gerontologist 18:541–546, 1978

Kilijanek TS, Drabek TE: Assessing long-term impacts of a natural disaster: a focus on the elderly. Gerontologist 19:555–566, 1979

Kulka RA, Schlenger WE, Fairbank JA, et al: Trauma and the Vietnam War Generation. New York, Brunner/Mazel, 1990

Leopold RL, Dillon H: Psycho-anatomy of a disaster: a long term study of post-traumatic neurosis in survivors of a marine explosion. Am J Psychiatry 120:913–921, 1963

Logue J, Hansen H, Struening E: Some indications of the long-term health effects of a natural disaster. Public Health Rep 96:67–79, 1981

Myers JK, Weissman MM, Tischler GL, et al: Six month prevalence of psychiatric disorders in three communities. Arch Gen Psychiatry 41:959–967, 1984

Norris FH, Phifer JF, Kaniasty KZ: Individual and community reactions to the Kentucky floods: findings from a longitudinal study of older adults, in Individual and Community Responses to Trauma and Disaster. Edited by Ursano R, McCaughey B, Fullerton C. Cambridge, England, Cambridge University Press, 1994, pp 378–400

Ollendick DG, Hoffmann M: Assessment of psychological reactions in disaster victims. Journal of Community Psychology 10:157–167, 1982

Price J: Some age-related effects of the 1974 Brisbane floods. Aust N Z J Psychiatry 12:55–58, 1978

Spitzer RL, Williams JW: Structured Clinical Interview for DSM-III: Non-patient Version (SCID-NP-11-1-6). New York, Biometrics Research Department, New York State Psychiatric Institute, 1986

Spitzer RL, Endicott J, Mesnikoff AM, et al: The Psychiatric Evaluation Form. New York, Biometrics Research Department, New York State Psychiatric Institute, 1968

Stern GM: The Buffalo Creek Disaster: The Story of the Survivors' Unprecedented Lawsuit. New York, Random House, 1976

Taylor AJW, Frazer AG: The stress of post-disaster body handling and victim identification work. Journal of Human Stress 8:4–12, 1982

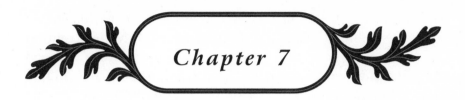

Chapter 7

Elder Maltreatment and Posttraumatic Stress Disorder

Marion Zucker Goldstein, M.D.

W e have learned to associate posttraumatic stress disorder (PTSD) with large-scale natural and human-made disasters. One such human-made disaster is the stress of victimization experienced in families, on the street, and in institutional settings. Considering the incidence and prevalence of violence experienced and witnessed in our society, these situations certainly amount to a "large scale."

The scale is even larger if we consider the repetitive and often unrelenting nature of these stressful experiences.

Domestic violence has finally come "out of the closet" and into the media as a social sickness. However, commonly held misperceptions still prevail: that domestic violence is rare, that it does not occur in "normal" relationships, and that it is a private matter. The emotional sequelae of such experiences in the context of PTSD have received considerably less attention than the drama of wars and natural disasters. More attention has been paid to the emotional sequelae of trauma suffered during childhood, adolescence, young adulthood, and midlife than to trauma suffered later in life. Furthermore, the late-life sequelae of having witnessed violence or having experienced neglect or exploitation earlier in life have also not received the needed attention. Greater awareness of child abuse occurred in the 1960s with mandatory reporting laws (Kempe et al. 1962), followed by spouse abuse reporting laws in the 1970s (Hilberman 1980; Straus et al. 1980), and finally elder abuse reporting laws in the 1980s (Burston 1975; Council on Scientific Affairs 1987; Goldstein 1989; Subcommittee on Health and Long Term Care of the Select Committee on Aging 1990).

Victimization by physical, emotional, and material abuse during each phase of the life cycle has been underdetected and underreported, leading to underrecognition and misdiagnosis of manifestations of PTSD at various times in the course of, or following, victimization.

Recent advances based on research findings in the conceptualization (American Psychiatric Association 1994; Davidson 1993) and treatment (Marmar 1993) of PTSD challenge us to weave this knowledge base into the clinical fabric of the practice of geriatric psychiatry as it pertains to victimization in the everyday lives of all too many of our ever-increasing number of elderly persons.

In this chapter, to focus attention on mistreatment experienced in late life, I consider the definitions, incidence, prevalence, and research findings of 1) elder abuse, neglect, and exploitation; 2) sequelae of victimization on mental status; 3) common defenses used by victimizer and provider of formal care that contribute to the high prevalence of underdetection; and 4) common profiles of elderly victims and those they depend on. The frail dependent elderly are a population at high risk for abuse, neglect, and exploitation. Those with dementia are at particular risk (Coyne et al. 1993; Moon and Williams 1993; Paveza et al. 1992).

Definition of Terms

Most researchers divide elder maltreatment into the categories of physical, material, and psychological abuse. A distinction is made between active abuse and passive neglect (Godkin et al. 1989). Physical abuse includes the infliction of physical pain or injury, slapping, sexual assault, bruising, physical coercion, confinement against one's will, molestation, cutting, burning, and physically restraining. Material abuse includes illegal or improper exploitation or use of funds or other resources or both. Psychological abuse is the infliction of mental anguish; calling a person derogatory names; treating a person with disrespect; and frightening, humiliating, intimidating, threatening, or isolating a person. Active neglect includes refusal or failure to fulfill caregiving obligations. It involves a conscious, intentional attempt to inflict physical or emotional distress on the elderly, deliberate abandonment, or denial of food or health-related services. Passive neglect is an unintentional refusal or failure to fulfill a caretaking obligation, thereby inflicting physical or emotional distress on the elderly. It often occurs because of inadequate knowledge, laziness, infirmity, or disputing the value of prescribed services. The problem of definitions has been reviewed extensively in the literature (Hudson 1991; Sellers et al. 1992) and continues to be a matter of concern and debate.

Epidemiology

Incidence and Prevalence: Community

The incidence and prevalence of elder maltreatment has been studied in several countries during the past 8 years. Both community and institutional populations have been investigated using a variety of methods and instruments.

A random sample community survey of 2,020 elderly persons in the Boston, Massachusetts, metropolitan area revealed a prevalence of 32 abused elderly per 1,000 population (Pille-mer and Finkelhor 1988). During the same time period as the study took place, Massachusetts reported an incidence rate of 1.8 per 1,000. Thus, only about 1 in every 14 cases had been officially reported. In this study, three-fifths of the perpetrators were spouses, one-fifth adult children, and one-fifth siblings, grandchildren, boarders, and others. Among the abusive adult children, sons outnumbered daughters 2:1.

These data differ from a 15-state data analysis of 1988, reported by the National Aging Resource Center on Elder Abuse.[1] This analysis revealed that 30% of abusive caregivers were adult children and 15% spouses.

A modified random sample telephone survey in Canada of 2,008 elderly persons living in private dwellings revealed that about 40 persons per 1,000 elderly population had experienced a serious form of maltreatment in their home (Podnieks 1992).

Incidence and Prevalence: Institutions

A survey of 577 staff of 57 nursing homes revealed that 36% of the sample had witnessed at least one incident of physical abuse in the preceding year, and 81% had observed at least one psychologically abusive incident (Pillemer and Moore 1989). In addition, 10% reported having committed at least one physically abusive act, and 40% reported having commit-ted at least one psychologically abusive act. The study took place prior to the 1987 Omnibus Budget Reconciliaton Act (OBRA) regulations, and observing excessive restraints was noted by 21% of the respondents and reported by 6%.

A small but controlled study of 51 caregivers of patients treated in geriatric respite services in Great Britain revealed that 45% of caregivers admitted to some form of abusive behaviors (Homer and Gilleard 1990).

---

[1] National Aging Resource Center on Elder Abuse, 810 First Street, NE, Suite 500, Washington, DC 20002-4205, (202) 682-2470.

Reporting of Maltreatment

Resistances to identification and reporting of abusive situations are multifaceted, have been studied in various settings and can be psychodynamically identified. Abusers and providers of formal care have psychological defenses in common such as denial, rationalization, and minimization. Respect for the older person's autonomy and family's privacy can create personal conflict for the professional provider of care.

Despite the fact that there are now mandatory reporting laws in 42 states and voluntary reporting laws in 8 states, many of the staff of 50 state health departments surveyed in 1991 were not aware of elder abuse reporting procedures (Anetzberger and Ehrlich 1991). Implementation of these laws lies with other state departments, and the results of this survey were felt to reflect a communication problem between the different state agencies.

A survey of emergency department personnel in Alabama revealed that reporting was hindered by dissatisfaction with response to reporting and fear of lengthy court hearings (Clark-Daniels et al. 1990).

Profile of the Maltreated Elderly

The profile of an elderly person who is at high risk for abuse is varied. These elderly often lack the opportunity and physical and mental ability to report abuses. Especially when the perpetrators of abuse are adult children, the victimized elderly person may desire to protect the children and may experience a great deal of embarrassment. Victimized parents who live at home often fear not being believed, reprisal, abandonment, and institutionalization. Victimized elderly are often women over age 75. Perceptions of elder abuse and help-seeking patterns have been found to vary among ethnic groups (Moon and Williams 1993).

Profile of Abusive Caregivers

The profiles of abusive caregivers are also very varied. These individuals require as much attention as the victim. Abusive caregivers have been identified as criminals, developmentally and/or mentally disabled individuals, substance abusers, gamblers, and chronic spouse abusers—but most frequently overstressed individuals who started out in their caregiving responsibilities with affection and dedication.

Posttraumatic Stress Disorder

With so many barriers to the identification and treatment of elder maltreatment, it is not surprising that identification and treatment of acute stress disorder and PTSD secondary to the trauma experienced often does not occur. Many symptoms that commonly present in the elderly—especially variations of sequelae of forgetfulness, anxiety, and depressed mood—are still mistakenly considered an inevitable consequence of the aging process by many primary care physicians. Even DSM-IV (American Psychiatric Association 1994), when it comes to diagnostic criteria for PTSD, alerts the researcher, student, teacher, and clinician only to a child's disorganization and agitated behavior following exposure to traumatic events in which a "person experienced, witnessed, or was confronted with an event or events that involved actual or threatened death or serious injury, or a threat to the physical integrity of self or others" (American Psychiatric Association 1994, p. 427). In the elderly maltreated person, the "intense fear, helplessness, or horror" (p. 428) can manifest itself also by "disorganized or agitated behavior" (p. 428) generally labeled as "confusion" at best and "old age" at worst.

The ways in which the traumatic event is persistently reexperienced are again only modified for children in DSM-IV and not for the older traumatized person. Especially in an older demented individual, the content of the reexperienced trauma may be expressed in the form of a delusion without ability to recall the actual facts. Manifestations of the trauma of neglect include malnutrition, dehydration, delirium, signs of inadequate or excessive hearing, and the absence of prosthetic aids where needed.

Although the abusive use of medications are excluded as a type of stressor (American Psychiatric Association 1994), this form of abuse in the elderly will require future reconsideration for inclusion in the stressor category. Manifestations of abuse of the use of medications, prescribed or over the counter, could include a state of delirium, memory impairment, agitation, lethargy, and self-neglect. Being "doped up," given a dose of medications suitable for a younger person, or given the wrong or excessive medication is often perceived as a severe trauma by elderly persons and occurs with considerable frequency in late life. Avoiding "activities, places, or people that arouse recollections of the trauma" (American Psychiatric Association 1994, p. 428) may manifest itself by avoiding the informal or formal provider of care. The feeling of life being over—"sense of a foreshortened future" (p. 428)—may be perceived as "normal" in an 80-year-old person by those unaware of the abuse or course of the aging process.

Control, isolation, and intimidation can foster the so well-known traumatic bonding of dependency on the abuser and avoidance of relationships with others. Effectiveness of intervention strategies will depend on improved assessments and identification of elder maltreatment as well as improved recognition of the varied manifestations of PTSD in the older population.

References

American Psychiatric Association: Diagnostic and Statistical Manual of Mental Disorders, 4th Edition. Washington, DC, American Psychiatric Association, 1994

Anetzberger C, Ehrlich P: Survey of state public health departments on procedures for reporting elder abuse. Public Health Rep 106:151–154, 1991

Burston GR: Granny battering. BMJ 36:592, 1975

Clark-Daniels CL, Daniels RS, Baumhover LA: Abuse and neglect of the elderly: are emergency department personnel aware of mandatory reporting laws? Ann Emerg Med 19:970–977, 1990

Council on Scientific Affairs: Report: American Medical Association: Elder Abuse and Neglect. JAMA 257:966–971, 1987

Coyne AC, Reichman WI, Berbig LJ: The relationship between dementia and elder abuse. Am J Psychiatry 150:643–646, 1993

Davidson J: Issues in the diagnosis of post traumatic stress disorder, in American Psychiatric Press Review of Psychiatry, Vol 12. Edited by Oldham JM, Riba MB, Tasman A. Washington, DC, American Psychiatric Press, 1993, pp 141–155

Godkin MA, Wolf RS, Pillemer KA: A case comparison analysis of elder abuse and neglect. Int J Aging Hum Dev 28:207–225, 1989

Goldstein MZ: Elder neglect, abuse and exploitation, in Family Violence: Emerging Issues of a National Crisis. Edited by Dickstein LJ, Nadelson CC. Washington, DC, American Psychiatric Press, 1989, pp 99–124

Hilberman E: Overview of the wife beater's wife reconsidered. Am J Psychiatry 137:1336–1347, 1980

Hudson MF: Elder mistreatment: a taxonomy with definitions by Delphi. Journal of Elder Abuse and Neglect 3:1–20, 1991

Homer AC, Gilleard C: Abuse of elder people by their cares. BMJ 301:1359–1362, 1990

Kempe CH, Silverman FN, Steele BF, et al: The battered child syndrome. JAMA 181:17–24, 1962

Marmar CR, Foy D, Kagan B, et al: An integrated approach for treating post traumatic stress, in American Psychiatric Press Review of Psychiatry, Vol 12. Edited by Oldham JM, Riba MB, Tasman A. Washington, DC, American Psychiatric Press, 1993, pp 239–272

Moon A, Williams O: Perceptions of elder abuse and help seeking pattern among African-American, Caucasian American and Korean-American elderly women. Gerontologist 33:386–395, 1993

Paveza GY, Cohen D, Eisdorfer C, et al: Severe family violence and Alzheimer's disease: prevalence and risk factors. Gerontologist 32:493–497, 1992

Pillemer K, Finkelhor D: The prevalence of elder abuse: a random sample survey. Gerontologist 28:51–57, 1988

Pillemer K, Moore DW: Abuse of patients in nursing homes: findings from a survey of staff. Gerontologist 29:314–319, 1989

Podnieks E: National survey of abuse of the elderly in Canada. Journal of Elder Abuse and Neglect 4:5–59, 1992

Sellers CS, Folts WE, Logan KM: Elder mistreatment: a multidimensional problem. Journal of Elder Abuse and Neglect 4:5–23, 1992

Straus MA, Gelles RJ, Steinmetz SK: Behind Closed Doors: Violence in American Families. New York, Doubleday, 1980

Subcommittee on Health and Long Term Care of the Select Committee on Aging: A Report of the Chairman of the Subcommittee on Health and Long Term Care of the Select Committee on Aging, House of Representatives: Elder Abuse: A Decade of Shame and Inaction (Comm Publ No 101–752). Washington, DC, U.S. Government Printing Office, 1990

Part III

Models of Stress in the Elderly

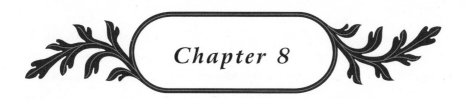

Chapter 8

The Impact of Ordinary Major and Small Negative Life Events on Older Adults

Charles A. Guarnaccia, Ph.D., and
Alex J. Zautra, Ph.D.

I n contrast to the extraordinary traumas examined in the rest of this book, the life experiences of most people are limited to ordinary negative events. These ordinary negative life events do not trigger posttraumatic stress disorder (PTSD), but they do both disrupt life and have an impact on mental health. In this chapter, we refer to research that relates ordinary negative events, coping efforts, and social support to the mental health of older adults. The effects of such ordinary negative events are illus-

The Arizona State University—Life Events and Aging Project was supported by National Institute on Aging Grant numbers NIA RO1 AG0-4924-01-02 and NIA RO1 AG0-4924-01-04 to Alex J. Zautra. The support of the National Institute on Aging is gratefully acknowledged.

trated with findings from a large gerontology research program. We do not provide an extensive review of the effects of negative events on older adults. Rather, the effects of a few common life events for older adults are presented to contrast the extraordinary life traumas discussed in the rest of this book.

Ordinary Negative Events of Older Adults

Major negative life events are often profound milestones for older adults. These negative occurrences include such major life disruptions as the death of a spouse, other relative, or close friend; a disabling illness; or institutionalization. Such events are common occurrences, although infrequent for any one individual. These major life events have a powerful effect on mental health (Markides and Cooper 1989). In contrast, the ordinary upsets of day-to-day existence include such occurrences as an argument with a family member, a minor illness, or a missed visit with a favorite grandchild. These small daily upsets (Kanner et al. 1981; Zautra et al. 1987) can also impact mental health.

The major negative events of later life can devastate older adults, even though these occurrences are well within the range of normal human experience. These events can cause long-lasting psychological distress, disrupt long-standing relationships, involve monumental life changes, require prolonged life readjustment, and even precipitate the onset of terminal decline for older adults. Among these events, the death of a spouse may be the most disturbing negative life event experienced by many older adults (Bowlby 1980; Osterweis et al. 1984; Stroebe and Stroebe 1987). A serious disabling illness is another common experience for older adults that, like conjugal bereavement, typically involves monumental life changes. The personal threat inherent in a major health decline may result in more long-term psychological devastation than the death of a spouse (Sinnot 1984–1985; Zautra et al. 1990). The death of a spouse and the onset of a serious illness or disability provide concrete examples of common major life stressors of later life.

Day-to-day negative experiences are benign frequent occurrences in comparison to the major negative events. These day-to-day negative events take the form of such minor upsets as a disagreement with a spouse, a restless night of fitful sleep, an unpleasant interaction with a rude salesperson, a day of minor pain, an unexpected auto repair expense, or an unpleasant visit with children or grandchildren. Although not life shattering, these small-event stressors increase psychological distress and lower psychological well-being of older adults (Kanner et al. 1981; Lewinsohn et al. 1985; Teri and Lewinsohn 1982; Zautra and Guarnaccia 1988; Zautra et al. 1989a, 1991).

Stress of Stressful Life Events

Systematic research on life stress dates to the animal analogue studies of Hans Selye (1956). Human stress and coping process has been examined by research over the past 25 years (Cohen 1988; Dohrenwend and Dohrenwend 1974, 1981a, 1981b; Holmes and Rahe 1967; Lazarus and Folkman 1984; Monroe 1982; Rabkin and Struening 1976; Thoits 1982). Life stress, indicated by the occurrence of events, provides a measure of the impact of the environment on individuals (Chiriboga 1989). This human research examines the relationship between life event stress and health outcomes. Following the lead of Holmes and Rahe (1967), event research with older adults first conceptualized major negative events as catastrophes. Within this catastrophe model, the same event (e.g., death of a spouse) was conceptualized as equivalent across individuals, with idiographic qualities being largely ignored (Chiriboga 1989). Current life event research views life stress as a person-environment transaction consisting of the stressor event, the environment, and the person along with the person's resources (Dohrenwend and Dohrenwend 1981a, 1981b; Lazarus and Folkman 1984). Life event research with older adults now takes this more complex view, examining the interplay of the stressor event within a specific environment; personal traits, perceptions, and actions; and available social support (Markides and Cooper 1989). Such nonevent factors add layers of complexity to a mixture of major and small negative life events. These nonevent components determine how the experience of an objectively similar event can differ. Personality traits and individual coping efforts are major person variables in this person-environment transaction. Personality factors can directly cause, or contribute to, a negative event (e.g., an irritable individual having an argument with a son- or daughter-in-law).

Personality traits can also affect the individual's response to an event and the individual's assessment of his or her ability to meet the demands of a stressor (e.g., a dependent older adult may ask a daughter or son to intervene to get a needed auto repair done at a garage). Coping responses, although influenced by stable personality factors, are also determined by qualities of the stressor event and available resources (Costa and McCrae 1989). In addition to this complex interaction among stressor event, personality, and coping efforts is coping efficacy, the individual's assessment of his or her success in coping (McCrae and Costa 1988; Zautra and Wrabetz 1991).

Social support has been added to this person-environment transactional model (Barrera 1986; Cohen and Wills 1985; Gottlieb 1983; Krause 1986). Social support refers to the emotional and instrumental assistance provided by individuals in a person's social network. Social support helps determine the relationship between the person-environment event transaction and mental health for older adults, although these effects are complex (Krause 1989; Thoits 1982). One of the primary ways that social support operates is as a stress buffer (Barrera

1988; Lin 1986; Wheaton 1985). Stress buffering occurs when social support reduces negative effects when life stress is high, but becomes less influential when life stress is low. As George (1989) pointed out, social support is particularly effective in reducing depression and depressive symptoms during times of high stress. She also noted that the issue is not whether life stress is injurious and social support provides protection against this injury, but under what specific conditions these injurious and protective influences occur and their mechanism of operation.

These constructs—the stressor event, the environment, the individual's traits, social support, and coping responses—all act together to determine how adults evaluate and are affected by major and small life event stressors. It is also worth noting that these relationships are likely not unidirectional. George (1989) commented on this complexity for the effects of social support. For example, social support may act to increase self-esteem and in this way reduce the relationship between life stress and depression (Krause 1987). Alternately, those with high self-esteem/self-efficacy may act to rally social support and thus reduce depressive outcome (Holahan and Holahan 1987).

Many of these factors operate for adults of any age. Life event stress for older adults also has elements of the role loss (George 1980) and life transitions (Perlin et al. 1981) that characterize later life. Negotiation of these changes determines successful adaptation to later life (Maddox and Campbell 1985). These changes are reflected in both the major and small negative events of later life. Major life events (e.g., widowhood, illness, institutionalization) and the small day-to-day occurrences that result are the way that the transitions of older adulthood are experienced. We now turn our attention to a research program that examines the relationship between two common negative major life events of later life (i.e., conjugal bereavement and physical disability) and daily life occurrences, mental health, social support, and personality factors.

The Life Events and Aging Project (LEAP)

Overview of the LEAP Study

The effects of ordinary major and small life events on older adults can be found in the results of the LEAP study (Zautra 1984, 1986). LEAP is a longitudinal study of high-risk community-dwelling older adults and matched control subjects. The high-risk conditions studied are two common uncontrollable major event stressors of later life: the death of a spouse and the onset of a functional disability due to a serious illness or injury.

Uncontrollable negative major life events were used to separate cause from effect within the LEAP study. Psychological state was removed as a cause of the major stressor event by using uncontrollable events, rather than stressors over which these older adults have causal influence. Conjugal bereavement and physical disability are important major life events to study, not only because they are common stressors of later life, but because their relationship with psychological state is unconfounded. By unconfounded, we mean that the causal relationship between the stressor event and outcome can be clearly understood because the possibility that psychological state has caused these uncontrollable events has been eliminated.[1] In this way we are able to study the effects of major life events in later life without becoming hopelessly lost in the

---

[1] Some may argue that the death of a spouse and, particularly, the onset of a physical disability may not be uncontrollable and may not be independent of preexisting psychological state. It is certainly the case that both of these events are likely influenced by a lifetime of health behaviors. This type of control is thus within the domain of a long-standing lifestyle rather than specific behaviors that intentionally cause a major event. By comparing the death of a spouse and the onset of a physical disability with major controllable events—such as retirement from a job, a move to a retirement community, divorce, (re)marriage, or another directly controllable change in social network or change in social role—the difference on this controllability dimension becomes clear.

reciprocal influences of events and psychological states on one another.

Concerning the sample, all LEAP participants were between the ages of 60 and 80 at the first interview in this longitudinal study. One-quarter of the LEAP participants, 61 older adults, suffered the death of a spouse in the 4–6 months before the study began. This subsample of "recently conjugally bereaved" was not physically disabled as judged by being below a cut score on an Instrumental Activities of Daily Living (IADL) scale (J. Q. Teresi, R. R. Golden, B. J. Gurland, D. E. Wilder, R. G. Bennett, Construct validity of indicator scales developed from the Comprehensive Assessment and Referral Evaluation Interviews Schedule, unpublished manuscript, 1983 [Available from The Center for Geriatrics, Columbia University]). Another quarter of the LEAP participants, 62 older adults, experienced the onset or exacerbation of a serious illness or injury during the 3 months before the study. This subsample of "disabled" participants had an associated reduction in physical ability as judged by being above the same IADL (Teresi et al., unpublished manuscript, 1983) cut score. These disabled persons had not been conjugally bereaved in the past 2 years. Thus, the recently conjugally bereaved and recently physically disabled were chosen to be mutually exclusive. Finally, 123 older adults were control subjects matched with the 61 conjugally bereaved and the 62 disabled groups for age, sex, and socioeconomic status. These 61 control subjects for the conjugally bereaved and 62 control subjects for the disabled were themselves neither recently conjugally bereaved nor functionally disabled. Thus, the control, conjugally bereaved, and disabled groups were mutually exclusive.

In the LEAP study, participants were interviewed once a month for 10 consecutive months by a trained older adult female interviewer. Following these 10 monthly interviews there was a 6-month follow-up interview (16 months after the initial interview). During each interview the older adult participants were questioned about major and small life events they had recently experienced. The PERI Major Life Events

Scale (Dohrenwend et al. 1978), modified for use with an older adult population (Zautra 1984, 1986), was used to measure major life stressors. The Older Adult-Inventory of Small Life Events (Zautra 1984, 1986; Zautra and Guarnaccia 1988; Zautra et al. 1986) measured desirable and undesirable small life events.[2] To measure mental health, we created an older adult version (Zautra et al. 1988a) of the combined Mental Health Inventory (Veit and Ware 1983), PERI Demoralization Composite (Dohrenwend et al. 1980), and the Bradburn Positive Affect Scale (Bradburn 1969). This older adult mental health measure consists of two major factors: psychological distress (consisting of anxiety/dread, depression, suicidal ideation, PERI anxiety, helplessness-hopelessness, and confused thinking subfactors) and psychological well-being (consisting of Mental Health Inventory positive affect, emotional ties, self-esteem, and Bradburn Positive Affect subfactors). During the first monthly interview, the 10th monthly interview, and the follow-up interview, social support network data were collected. Using these measures, the LEAP study examined the impact of the two common uncontrollable adaptive challenges of later adult life—conjugal bereavement and physical disability—on the mental health and daily lives of older adults.

Effects of Major Life Events

The effects of these two major stressors—death of a spouse and physical disability—is reflected in group differences. Differences between bereaved, disabled, and control groups are caused by the two uncontrollable life stressors rather than any

[2] The Inventory of Small Life Events and the Older Adult-Inventory of Small Life Events are available from Alex J. Zautra, Ph.D., Department of Psychology, Arizona State University, Tempe, AZ 85287-1104. Like the PERI Major Life Events Scale (Dohrenwend et al. 1978), the Inventory of Small Life Events (Zautra et al. 1986) and the Older Adult-Inventory of Small Life Events (Zautra and Guarnaccia 1988) include ratings of event control, causation, and required readjustment.

preexisting psychological differences as these selected stressors are beyond the individuals' direct control. Table 8–1 compares demographic/group selection and personality variables across groups at the first interview. There are a number of differences between groups. Differences on percentage widowed and IADL scores result directly from the group's selection criteria for the conjugally bereaved and disabled. Marginally lower average yearly income and percentage employed for disabled participants are also related to their poorer physical health. One of the two remaining differences, the disabled and bereaved participants being less extroverted than control subjects, may be related to their recent life stressors. The other remaining difference, the disabled participants being less well educated than either the bereaved or control groups, may be less a psychological process and more related to the protective influence on health of being of higher socioeconomic status (Krause 1990).

Concerning psychological distress, the disabled participants were both more anxious and more depressed than the control group. The bereaved participants were likewise more depressed than the control group, but were no more anxious. The disabled participants, in general, displayed more psychological disturbance than the bereaved group. The disabled participants had lower levels of both positive affect and self-esteem than did the control group. The bereaved participants showed no such widespread differences or trend toward generally poor adjustment. These findings suggest that the disabled participants have been more negatively impacted by their stressor than have the bereaved participants. The death of a spouse, although precipitating a life transition, seemed to leave the bereaved participants with their self-concept intact. The disabled group, perhaps because of the more personal nature of their stressor (i.e., the failure of their own physical being), appeared to have fewer psychological resources left to cope with the demands of their role transition (George 1980; Perlin et al. 1981). This can be understood in terms of the likely assault on self-concept of a loss in personal functional

Table 8–1. Comparisons among groups at the first interview

Variable	Participant group (mean)			F	χ^2
	Disabled (n = 61)	Bereaved (N = 62)	Control subjects (N = 123)		
Demographic/group selection variables					
Age (years)	71.6	69.3	71.0	1.63	1.17
Gender (% female)	78.3	82.5	75.6		1.55
Minority group status (%)	1.7	0.0	2.4		12.05**
Completed high school (%)	62.5ᵃ	84.1ᵇ	77.9ᵇ		
Occupational status-self[1]	4.57	4.50	4.38	.17	
Occupational status-spouse[1]	4.11	4.11	4.37	.59	
Average annual income ($)	11,666ᵃ	14,960ᵇ	13,728ᵇ	2.66*	
Yearly income under $9,000 (%)	47.4	28.6	33.1	1.61	5.12*
Employed (%)	1.7ᵃ	11.7ᵇ	11.3ᵇ		
Number of children	3.13	2.39	2.52	2.27	
Marital status					
Widowed (%)	41.7ᵃ	100ᵇ	36.0ᵃ		78.60***
Married (%)	40.3ᵃ	0ᵇ	48.8ᵃ		44.13***

IADL scores	13.4[a]	1.28[b]	1.62[b]	223.76***
Personality variables				
Neuroticism	1.40	1.42	1.35	2.04
Extroversion	1.64[a]	1.66[a]	1.74[b]	3.83**

Note. Values on the same row with an "a" superscript are significantly different from those with a "b" superscript.
[1]Occupational status is based on a 7-point rating scale (A. B. Hollingshead: Four factor index of social status, unpublished manuscript, Yale University, Department of Sociology, New Haven, 1975). A rating of 4 corresponds to clerical and sales work. A rating of 5 corresponds to skilled manual work.
*$P < .10$. **$P < .05$. ****$P < .001$.

ability and the life-threatening nature of a serious illness for older adults (Zautra et al. 1989a).

A serious physical disability being more psychologically destructive than the death of a spouse held up over the course of the 10 monthly interviews. Bereaved participants showed improvements over time with successively less depression and higher positive affect. In contrast, disabled participants showed only modest improvement in positive affect and continued to show elevations in depression. Disabled participants still remained at levels of psychological adjustments below that of control participants (Reich et al. 1989) after the 10 months. These results, which suggests the disabled participants are worse off than the conjugally bereaved participants, is in opposition to assumptions of early life stress research done with the Social Readjustment Rating Scale (Holmes and Rahe 1967). This scale, developed for the general adult population, suggests that the death of a spouse nearly tops the list of major stressors, being second only to the death of a child.

The difficultly disabled participants have in their psychological accommodation to this stressor can be brought into clearer focus. By evaluating IADL, psychological distress, and psychological well-being measures for the disabled participants, Zautra et al. (1989b) found that the individual's level of activity limitation predicted psychological outcome. Those disabled participants classified as more impaired experienced higher levels of anxiety, suicidal ideation, and general psychological distress than moderately disabled participants (Zautra et al. 1989b). This relationship between level of disability and psychological status was stable across time.

When comparing bereaved and disabled participants over the course of the 10 months, the bereaved participants maintained their superior psychological status. The bereaved participants showed greater reduction in psychological distress and greater increase in psychological well-being over the 10 months than did the disabled participants. These changes in the psychological functioning of bereaved and disabled participants suggest that the death of a spouse is an stressor from which most can recover. In contrast, the onset of a health problem with a loss in functional ability has longer-lasting implications for the affective states of older adults (Reich et al. 1989). Within the disabled participants, level of disability directly predicted level of psychological impairment (Zautra et al. 1989b).

Effects of Small Life Events

Besides the effects of the two major stressor events that defined group differences, the disabled, bereaved, and control participants led eventful daily lives. At the first interview, the 246 participants (i.e., 61 bereaved, 62 disabled, 123 control subjects) experienced an average of 13.5 desirable small events (e.g., visited grandchildren, went out with friends), 4.0 undesirable small events (e.g., criticized by friend), and 5.3 small health problems (e.g., began a day with physical discomfort) in the previous month. These daily life event reports predicted both psychological distress and psychological well-being across these three groups. Small desirable and undesirable events and health problems accounted for 15% of the variance in the prediction of psychological distress and 19% of the variance in the prediction of psychological well-being, even when neuroticism was controlled to account for the variation in psychological distress and well-being due to personality factors.

Even though daily events were predictive of both negative and positive psychological status across all participants, there were notable differences in event reports across the three participant groups. As might be expected, when the disabled and bereaved participants were compared with control subjects, differences in the occurrence of small events were noted that relate to the previously experienced uncontrollable major stressors. For example, the disabled participants reported significantly more health symptoms, health discomforts, and health promotion activities (e.g., saw a physician) than matched control subjects. As would be expected, due to poorer health, the disabled participants also reported engaging in fewer desirable small events than other participants.

By collecting expert ratings of the probable cause of the small life events, we were able to examine these differences in more detail. Using these expert ratings, the nature of the increased number of undesirable daily events experienced by the disabled participants fit the picture that has thus far been painted. The disabled participants experienced more externally caused (i.e., not directly caused by the participant) undesirable small events (e.g., minor physical pain) than did the bereaved participants, but not more internally caused (i.e., directly caused by the participant) undesirable small events (e.g., critical of family member) (Zautra et al. 1988b). These small-event findings suggest that day-to-day life for disabled older adults may be less enjoyable than for peers, even conjugally bereaved peers. These findings suggest that the disabled participants are not in control of much of the negative occurrences that color their day-to-day lives (Zautra et al. 1989a).

In longitudinal analyses for all subjects, Zautra et al. (1991) examined the best predictors of daily life events. Using a causal model, they found that the major stressors—conjugal bereavement and physical disability—played a role in daily event occurrences. Personality variables played only a minor role in the prediction of these daily events. The best predictor of future events was previous event occurrence; that is, the occurrence of daily events was found to be stable over time.

This suggests that on a day-to-day and month-to-month level, small daily occurrences in the lives of older adults stand as ongoing themes, with the reverberations of major life changes being felt through ongoing daily occurrences. This certainly seems to be the case for the disabled participants in this research. The daily lives of these disabled older adults revolve around their physical health status. Event reports suggest that the bereaved participants are also forced to focus on their new roles, but in a way that may be less psychologically taxing. We were able to provide some detail to the daily lives of these older adults by examining the small day-to-day events, as well as the major stressors, of these older adults. In this way, stress and coping research can extend its understanding of how common major stressors of later adulthood reverberate through the daily experiences of these older adults.

Resistance Resources in Times of Stress

The social support networks of these participants were also examined. Finch et al. (1989) found the factor structure of social ties to be similar, but not identical, among the three groups. As both positive and negative social ties were evaluated, this study looked at the effects of both supportive and nonsupportive social network associations on psychological distress and psychological well-being. Finch et al. found that positive social ties (i.e., traditional social support) were predictive of higher levels of psychological well-being, whereas negative social ties (i.e., social relationships that have some significant negative aspects) were predictive of both higher levels of psychological distress and lower levels of psychological well-being. Interestingly, positive social ties and negative social ties were found to be independent of one another. This suggests that both the positive and negative aspects of social relationships must be assessed to get a complete picture of how these two forces impact on the mental health of older adults.

Zautra and Wrabetz (1991) evaluated the coping efficacy of the older adults in this study who, during the course of the 10 monthly interviews, experienced either a major health problem (e.g., serious illness got worse) or a social loss (e.g., death of a close friend). In a cross-sectional analysis, Zautra and Wrabetz found that those who were actively engaged in attempting to cope with these health downturns and social losses showed lower psychological distress. A longitudinal analysis supports the same finding of lower psychological distress for those who were actively coping with a social loss. Thus the active attempt to cope with major uncontrollable stressor events is also involved in determining the psychological effects of events. These findings agree with George (1989), who mentioned that life events have fewer negative consequences if the individual has higher self-efficacy.

Because the LEAP study collected longitudinal data, Guarnaccia (1990) was able to investigate whether the bereaved participants were assisted by their bereavement experience when coping with subsequently major losses. The bereaved participants were less centrally affected by a subsequent loss event (e.g., the death of a close friend) than were married control subjects. This improvement in coping with loss may be a stress inoculation effect caused by the conjugal bereavement. Guarnaccia also found that the conjugal bereavement experience influenced coping with later thematically similar events, independent of personality characteristics such as neuroticism. Those bereaved participants who coped better with their bereavement had fewer negative changes due to subsequent thematically similar loss events. Thus, the impact of events depended on the resolution of past similar problems and not personality characteristics.

Summary

As can be seen in this overview of the findings from the LEAP study, major life event stressors do not act independently to predict mental health outcome. Although uncontrollable major negative events of later life, such as the death of a spouse or the onset of a physical disability, have a powerful influence on determining subsequent psychological state, qualities of those affected, their day-to-day lives, their social networks, and their perceptions of their own coping all act together to determine their subsequent psychological distress and well-being. We hope that this chapter highlights some of the important person and environment factors that should be accounted for whether older adults are coping with normative life events or extraordinary life traumas.

The longitudinal design of the LEAP study allowed us to judge the effects of two major uncontrollable stressors on subsequent life events and on psychological distress and well-being. We were also able to assess the effects of social support and other variables on the process of adaptation to these challenges of later life. In keeping with suggestions for gerontological research (George 1989; Markides and Cooper 1989), the LEAP study, besides assessing the effects of single major stressors, such as widowhood, also includes other measures of life stress. The LEAP study, besides being a longitudinal study that collected major life event and mental health data in monthly interviews, also measured daily life upset as well as negative social support. Research interviews of this detail, although difficult to complete, provide a more comprehensive picture of the ongoing lives of older adults than is typically available from research.

The various influences noted throughout this chapter all contribute to the stressful nature of negative life events. This list of factors may still be lacking elements that will become noteworthy in future research with older adults. For instance, the role losses and transitions of later life may result in a decrease in the goal-motivated skill/challenge activity of adult daily life. In this way, role losses may cause an unwanted deprivation of the desired flow of life (Csikszentmihalyi and Csikszentmihalyi 1988). It is also likely that the thematic meaning of major events for older adults may also hold meaning beyond the objective event. Concerning almost trivial daily upsets, Lazarus (1978) wrote

> The shoelace might break, but a major part of the psychological stress created thereby is the implication that one cannot control one's life, that one is helpless in the face of the most stupid of trivialities, or even worse, that one's own inadequacies have made the obstacle occur in the first place. (p. 8)

This suggests that when small, seemingly trivial, events cluster together, they may have a powerful effect on how individuals view their lives. Day (1981, 1989) reported that life events preceding acute schizophrenic episodes have an ordinary day-to-day quality.

With this chapter and its examples from the LEAP study, we hope to highlight the need to measure both major and small life occurrences when attempting to understand life stress. In this way, gerontological researchers will know how major stressors of later life reverberate in the day-to-day upsets of older adults. Everyday life is an important, but neglected, source of stress in the lives of older adults; it cannot continue to be ignored in life event research. The detail provided by daily life transactions is needed to understand both older adults who have experienced a common but painful major stressor of later life and older adults who have experienced the effects of trauma well beyond the range of normal human experience.

The finding of subsequent coping being predicted by previous success, independent of personality traits (Guarnaccia 1990), may be of use when evaluating the effects of extraordinary trauma on PTSD. It may be beneficial to study the negative small life events of those with PTSD. Events associated with PTSD symptoms may form a yet undiscovered link between everyday life and past unresolved problems. This may operate through the thematic content of events. An understanding of this relationship beyond the bounds of PTSD to include general stress and coping research may tie these two fields together more closely. This would benefit life stress theory by providing data from extraordinary stressful events. PTSD theory would likely advance as it could be modeled as an extension of a commonly occurring life process. Thus, life stress and PTSD theory and research would advance if both could be understood by a unified conceptual model.

References

Barrera M: Distinctions between social support concepts, measures, and models. Am J Community Psychol 14:413–445, 1986

Barrera M: Models of social support and life stress, in Life Events and Psychological Functioning: Theoretical and Methodological Issues. Edited by Cohen LH. Newbury Park, CA, Sage, 1988, pp 211–236

Bowlby J: Attachment and Loss, Vol 3: Loss: Sadness and Depression. New York, Basic Books, 1980

Bradburn N: The Structure of Psychological Well-Being. Chicago, IL, Adline, 1969

Chiriboga DA: The measurement of stress exposure in later life, in Aging, Stress and Health. Edited by Markides KS, Cooper CL. New York, Wiley, 1989, pp 241–268

Cohen LH (ed): Life Events and Psychological Functioning: Theoretical and Methodological Issues. Newbury Park, CA, Sage, 1988

Cohen S, Wills T: Stress, social support, and the buffering hypothesis. Psychol Bull 98:310–357, 1985

Costa PT, McCrae RR: Personality, stress, and coping: some lessons from a decade of research, in Aging, Stress and Health. Edited by Markides KS, Cooper CL. New York, Wiley, 1989, pp 241–268

Csikszentmihalyi M, Csikszentmihalyi IS (eds): Optimal Experience: Studies of Flow in Consciousness. New York, Cambridge University Press, 1988

Day R: Life events and schizophrenia: the triggering hypothesis. Acta Psychiatr Scand 64:97–122, 1981

Day R: Schizophrenia, in Life Events and Illness. Edited by Brown GW, Harris TO. New York, Guilford, 1989, pp 113–138

Dohrenwend BS, Dohrenwend BP (eds): Stressful Life Events: Their Nature and Effects. New York, Wiley, 1974

Dohrenwend BS, Dohrenwend BP: Socioenvironmental factors, stress, and psychopathology, part 2: hypotheses about stress processes linking social class to various types of psychopathology. Am J Community Psychol 9:146–159, 1981a

Dohrenwend BS, Dohrenwend BP (eds): Stressful Life Events and Their Contexts. New York, Prodist, 1981b

Dohrenwend BS, Krasnoff L, Askenasy AR, et al: Exemplification of a method for scaling life events: the PERI life events scale. J Health Soc Behav 19:205–229, 1978

Dohrenwend BP, Shrout PE, Egri G, et al: Non-specific psychological distress and other dimensions of psychopathology. Arch Gen Psychiatry 37:1229–1236, 1980

Finch JF, Okun MA, Barrera M Jr, et al: Positive and negative social ties among older adults: measurement models and the prediction of psychological distress and well-being. Am J Community Psychol 17:585–605, 1989

George LK: Role Transitions in Later Life. Monterey, CA, Brooks/Cole, 1980

George LK: Stress, social support, and depression over the life-course, in Aging, Stress and Health. Edited by Markides KS, Cooper CL. New York, Wiley, 1989, pp 241–268

Gottlieb B: Social Support Strategies: Guidelines for Mental Health Practice. Newbury Park, CA, Sage, 1983

Guarnaccia CA: An alternate perspective on the effects of conjugal bereavement and general fateful loss: stress inoculation. Dissertation Abstracts International 52:517B, 1990

Holahan CK, Holahan CJ: Self-efficacy, social support, and depression in aging: a longitudinal analysis. J Gerontol 42:65–68, 1987

Holmes TH, Rahe RH: The social readjustment rating scale. J Psychosom Res 11:213–218, 1967

Kanner AD, Coyne JC, Schaeffer C, et al: Comparison of two modes of stress measurement: daily hassles and uplifts versus major life events. J Behav Med 4:1–39, 1981

Krause N: Social support, stress, and well-being among older adults. J Gerontol 41:512–519, 1986

Krause N: Chronic strain, locus of control, and distress in older adults. Psychol Aging 2:375–382, 1987

Krause N: Issues of measurement and analysis in studies of social support, aging and health, in Aging, Stress and Health. Edited by Markides KS, Cooper CL. New York, Wiley, 1989, pp 241–268

Krause N: Illness behavior in later life, in Handbook of Aging and the Social Sciences. Edited by Binstock RH, George LK. New York, Academic Press, 1990, pp 227—244

Lazarus RS: The stress and coping paradigm. Paper presented at a conference organized by Carl Eisdorfer et al. on "Critical Evaluation of Behavioral Paradigm for Psychiatric Science," Gleneden Beach, OR, 1978

Lazarus RS, Folkman S: Stress, Appraisal, and Coping. New York, Spring Publishing, 1984

Lin N: Modeling the effects of social support, in Social Support, Life Events, and Depression. Edited by Lin N, Dean A, Ensel W. New York, Academic Press, 1986, pp 173–209

Lewinsohn PM, Mermelstein RM, Alexader C, et al: The Unpleasant Events Schedule: a scale for the measurement of aversive events. J Clin Psychol 41:483–498, 1985

Maddox GL, Campbell RT: Scope, concepts, and methods in the study of aging, in Handbook of Aging and the Social Sciences, 2nd Edition. Edited by Binstock RH, Shanas E. New York, Van Nostrand Reinhold, 1985, pp 3–31

Markides KS, Cooper CL (eds): Aging, Stress and Health. New York, Wiley, 1989

McCrae RR, Costa PT: Personality, coping and effectiveness in an adult sample. J Pers 54:385–405, 1988

Monroe SM: Life events assessment: current practices, emerging trends. Clinical Psychology Review 2:435–453, 1982

Osterweis M, Solomom F, Green M (eds): Bereavement: Reactions, Consequences, and Care. Washington, DC, National Academy Press, 1984

Perlin LI, Lieberman MA, Menaghan EG, et al: The stress process. J Health Soc Behav 22:337–356, 1981

Rabkin JG, Struening EL: Life events, stress, and illness. Science 194:1013–1020, 1976

Reich JW, Zautra AJ, Guarnaccia CA: Effects of disability and bereavement on the mental health and recovery of older adults. Psychol Aging 4:57–65, 1989

Selye H: The Stress of Life. New York, McGraw-Hill, 1956

Sinnot JD: Stress, health, and mental health symptoms of older adult men and women. Int J Aging Hum Dev 20:123–132, 1984–1985

Stroebe W, Stroebe MS: Bereavement and Health: The Psychological and Physical Consequences of Partner Loss. New York, Cambridge University Press, 1987

Teri L, Lewinsohn PM: Modification of the Pleasant and Unpleasant Events Schedules for use with the elderly. J Consult Clin Psychol 50:444–445, 1982

Thoits PA: Conceptual, methodological, and theoretical problems in studying social support as a buffer against life stress. J Health Soc Behav 23:145–159, 1982

Veit CT, Ware JE: The structure of psychological distress and well-being in general populations. J Consult Clin Psychol 51:730–742, 1983

Wheaton B: Models of the stress-buffering functions of coping and social support. J Health Soc Behav 26:352–364, 1985

Zautra AJ: Life events and demoralization in the elderly, Grant 1 NIA RO1 AG04924-01. Washington, DC, National Institute on Aging, 1984

Zautra AJ: Life events and demoralization in the elderly, Grant 2 NIA RO1 AG04924-03. Washington, DC, National Institute on Aging, 1986

Zautra AJ, Guarnaccia CA: Research inventory of major and small life events for older adults. Paper presented at the 41st annual meeting of the Gerontological Society of America, San Francisco, CA, November, 1988

Zautra AJ, Wrabetz AB: Coping success and its relationship to psychological distress for older adults. J Pers Soc Psychol 61:801–810, 1991

Zautra AJ, Guarnaccia CA, Dohrenwend BP: Measuring small life events. Am J Community Psychol 14:629–655, 1986

Zautra AJ, Guarnaccia CA, Reich JW, et al: The contribution of small events to stress and distress, in Life Events and Psychological Functioning: Theoretical and Methodological Issues. Edited by Cohen LH. Newbury Park, CA, Sage, 1987, pp 123–148

Zautra AJ, Guarnaccia CA, Reich JW: The factor structure of mental health measures for older adults. J Consult Clin Psychol 56:514–519, 1988a

Zautra AJ, Guarnaccia CA, Carothers B: Measuring small events of older adults. Paper presented at the 41st annual meeting of the Gerontological Society of America, San Francisco, CA, November 1988b

Zautra AJ, Guarnaccia CA, Reich JW: The effects of daily life events on negative affective states, in Anxiety and Depression: Distinctive and Overlapping Features. Edited by Kendall PC, Watson D. New York, Academic Press, 1989a, pp 225–251

Zautra AJ, Maxwell BM, Reich JW: Relationship among physical impairment, distress, and well-being in older adults. J Behav Med 12:543–557, 1989b

Zautra AJ, Reich JW, Guarnaccia CA: Some everyday life consequences of disability and bereavement for older adults. J Pers Soc Psychol 59:550–561, 1990

Zautra AJ, Finch JF, Reich JW, et al: Predicting the everyday life events of older adults. J Pers 59:507–538, 1991

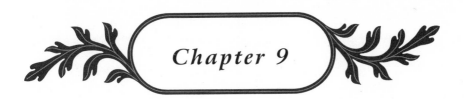

Chapter 9

Age Differences in Physiological Responses to Stress

Maya McNeilly, Ph.D., and
Norman B. Anderson, Ph.D.

In this section, we provide an overview of selected, representative studies of age differences in physiological responses to stress. Our objectives are 1) to describe the theoretical basis for stress-reactivity research, its utility in predicting disease, and the experimental paradigms used in this area; 2) to summarize results from research on physiological changes with aging and responses to stress; 3) to present conceptual and methodological issues important in conducting biobehavioral research with the

Portions of this chapter are based on an earlier review of sociodemographic aspects of physiological responses to stress (N. B. Anderson and McNeilly 1991).

elderly; 4) to discuss clinical applications of research on stress responsivity in the elderly; and 5) to suggest directions for future investigation.

Stress Reactivity: Rationale and Methodology

The theoretical basis underlying research in stress reactivity is that excessive physiological changes that may occur in response to stressors may contribute to the development of cardiovascular disease. Although the exact mechanisms by which this process occurs have yet to be specified, it is believed that exposure to stressors activates the sympathetic nervous system and hypothalamic-pituitary-adrenal axis, resulting in physiological changes that exceed the body's metabolic needs. These changes include increases in heart rate, blood pressure, perspiration, and the release of neuroendocrine substances. Over time, the repeated exposure to stress and excessive physiological arousal leads to autonomic nervous system (ANS) dysregulation and may result in diseases such as hypertension (Folkow 1989; Folkow et al. 1958; Matthews et al. 1986; Obrist 1981). For a more in-depth discussion of the reactivity hypothesis and the various physiological mechanisms by which stress-induced reactivity and disease may be linked, the reader is referred elsewhere (Manuck et al. 1990).

Support for the reactivity hypothesis is provided by studies with both animals and humans. In mice, rats, and dogs, for example, territorial conflict, residential crowding, disruptions in social status, and exposure to chronic stressors have been shown to produce exaggerated stress-induced pressor responses. These exaggerated responses were observed to precede the development of sustained high blood pressure (Hallback and Folkow 1974; Henry and Cassel 1969; Henry et al. 1975; Lundin and Thoren 1982).

Among humans, research has indicated that ANS reactivity to exercise, the cold pressor, and mental arithmetic tasks may predict hypertension development (Borghi et al. 1986; Jackson et al. 1983; Menkes et al. 1989; Pickering and Gerin 1990; Wood et al. 1984). In these studies, greater reactivity was associated with the later onset of hypertension. In a study noted for its methodological strengths (Menkes et al. 1989), researchers studied 910 white male medical students before and during the cold pressor test. After controlling for numerous potential confounding factors such as age at study entry, Quetelet index, cigarette smoking, pretest systolic blood pressure, and parental or maternal history of hypertension, it was observed that systolic blood pressure reactivity to the cold pressor test significantly predicted hypertension development 20–36 years later. Menkes et al. noted that the excess risk associated with systolic blood pressure reactivity became apparent only when subjects had aged approximately 20 years and was most apparent among those becoming hypertensive before age 45.

In a study using a mental arithmetic stressor, Borghi et al. (1986) found that among borderline hypertensive persons, diastolic blood pressure reactivity and recovery from the mental arithmetic task were significant predictors of sustained hypertension after 5 years. Those persons who exhibited greater reactivity and who had recovery pressures at least 6% above baseline levels were at greatest risk for developing sustained hypertension.

Furthermore, laboratory studies have shown that young and middle-age whites and blacks with established or borderline hypertension show cardiovascular and neuroendocrine hyperreactivity compared with subjects with normal blood pressure (Fredrikson et al. 1982; Hollenberg et al. 1981; Light and Sherwood 1989; Steptoe et al. 1984). A number of other studies have shown that whites with a parental history of hypertension show greater cardiovascular responses compared with the offspring of normotensive persons (Ditto 1986; Jorgensen and Houston 1981; Manuck and Proietti 1982).

Although these studies suggest that exaggerated stress reactivity may predict the later development of disease among younger individuals, not all studies support these findings (Barnett et al. 1963; Borghi et al. 1986; Ditto 1986; Durel et al. 1989; Eich and Jacobensen 1967; Harlan et al. 1964). Because of this, the reactivity hypothesis remains controversial. It should be noted, however, that many of these negative studies suffer from a number of methodological weaknesses including inadequate sample sizes, short duration follow-up, or inappropriate assessment of reactivity (Manuck et al. 1990).

Manuck et al. (1990) noted that autonomic reactivity may be linked to hypertension development in several ways. One way is that repeated increases in ANS activity may lead to augmented peripheral resistance and structural changes in the arterial walls, thereby directly contributing to the pathogenesis of hypertension (Folkow et al. 1958). Alternatively, a "diasthesis-stress" model predicts that autonomic reactivity may cause hypertension, but only if this response is frequently elicited over an extended period of time and only in individuals who have a biological predisposition to exaggerated reactivity. Those who experience repeated ANS arousals more frequently are thought to be at greater risk for developing hypertension. Yet another way in which autonomic reactivity may be linked to hypertension is thought to be through its interaction with other risk factors, such as dietary sodium (D. E. Anderson et al. 1983; Manuck et al. 1990). Lastly, ANS reactivity in and of itself may not be pathogenic, but may serve only as a risk marker predicting subsequent hypertension.

In a typical stress-reactivity experiment, physiological responses are recorded from the subject during an initial resting baseline period, during exposure to the stressor, and during recovery from the stressor. The magnitude as well as the pattern of physiological changes from resting to stress-induced and recovery levels of ANS activity provide useful information to researchers and clinicians. Ordinarily, the larger the response, the more significance it is thought to have relative to the pathogenesis or maintenance of disease. The patterns of cardiovascular and neuroendocrine responses, on the other hand, enable investigators to learn more about the nature of ANS arousal occurring in response to a stressor. For example, by examining the pattern of ANS responses, researchers may infer whether the changes are predominantly vascular or cardiac adrenergically mediated, or sympathetically versus parasympathetically mediated.

Tasks

A variety of challenging psychological, behavioral, and physical tasks have been utilized to assess stress reactivity in older and younger individuals. These have included cognitive, neuromotor, or behavioral tasks such as mental arithmetic, competitive and noncompetitive reaction time tasks, video games, insoluble anagrams, mirror tracing, the Stroop Color-Word task, and speech delivery. Challenges of a more physical nature have included the cold pressor task (hand or foot immersion and the forehead cold pressor), handgrip (dynamometer), orthostatic stress (head-up tilt or moving from a sitting to standing position), and physical exercise.

Studies have demonstrated that certain tasks produce different patterns of cardiovascular and neuroendocrine responses. For example, tasks such as mental arithmetic and video games have been shown to elicit a pattern of increased heart rate, stroke volume, cardiac output, and blood pressure. Other stressors such as the forehead cold pressor task and mirror tracing tend to elicit a pattern of decreased heart rate or attenuated heart increases, and increased vasoconstriction, peripheral resistance, and blood pressure. Utilizing tasks such as these allow investigators indirectly to examine patterns of adrenergic activity in the elderly.

Populations

Recent years have witnessed an increasing interest in identifying race and gender differences in stress reactivity in the young. This has been in part an attempt to determine whether these differences might assist in explaining the race and gender differences in prevalence rates of cardiovascular disease. This effort, however, has not been paralleled in studies of stress reactivity among the elderly. In fact, virtually all studies of reactivity in the elderly have included only white participants or failed to report the race of the subjects. Similarly, most reactivity research with the elderly has been conducted among males, with relatively little research directed specifically at women. Because studies suggest that race and gender play important roles in determining the magnitude and pattern of reactivity to stress in young adults, we include these data in our discussions of stress-induced physiological responses among the elderly, with the caveat that these effects may or may not hold true for older individuals.

Summary of Results From Studies on Aging and Stress Reactivity

Measurement of physiological responses to stress among the elderly has been used to identify physiological changes that occur with normal healthy aging in response to challenge and to determine and characterize ANS dysregulation that may occur with pathological aging. The main physiological systems that have been most extensively studied in stress-reactivity research include blood pressure (systolic and diastolic), heart rate, electrodermal activity, neuroendocrine responses, and alpha- and beta-adrenergic receptor function. In the following paragraphs, we briefly describe these response systems and their measurement and discuss age-related changes in these modalities at rest and in response to stress. For a more thorough review of the ANS and its measurement in psychophysiological studies, a number of excellent texts are available (e.g., Cacioppo and Petty 1983; Coles et al. 1986; Hassett 1978; Schneiderman et al. 1989; Stern et al. 1980).

Age Effects on Heart Rate

Heart rate, the speed at which the heart pumps, is usually measured as the number of beats-per-minute. In most stress-reactivity experiments, heart rate is digitally recorded by an automated monitor or measured as "R" waves recorded by electrocardiogram.

Epidemiologic and laboratory studies indicate that resting heart rate generally decreases with age and that the stress-induced increases in heart rate are attenuated in older compared with younger individuals (Faucheux et al. 1983; Finch 1977; Jose 1966; Kohn 1977). For example, investigations using both beta- and alpha-adrenergic agonist challenges have consistently demonstrated that older individuals show smaller heart rate increases relative to younger individuals. These decreases in heart rate are believed to reflect age-related changes in the sympathetic nervous system, which include a decrease in beta-adrenergic activity and sensitivity (Bertel et al. 1980; Buhler 1983; Dillon et al. 1980; Fleisch 1980; Lakatta and Yin 1982; van Brummelen et al. 1981; Vestal et al. 1979).

Similarly, studies employing a variety of behavioral, rather than pharmacologic, challenges have also indicated that in response to challenges such as cold exposure (Wagner and Horvath 1985), reaction time tasks (Gintner et al. 1986), isometric exercise (Goldstraw and Warren 1985; Matthews and Stoney 1988; Palmer et al. 1978), aerobic exercise (Fleg et al. 1985; Sato et al. 1981), orthostatic stress (Goldstein and Shapiro 1990; Palmer et al. 1978), and cognitive challenges (Barnes et al. 1982; Matthews and Stoney 1988), older individuals show smaller heart rate increases in response to stress compared with younger individuals.

Gender and age effects on heart rate. In general, both epidemiologic and laboratory studies indicate that females have faster resting heart rates and show greater increases in stress-induced heart rates relative to males (Bell et al. 1968; Collins and Frankenhaeuser 1978; McAdoo et al. 1990). Investigators have attributed this to the fact that females have smaller hearts than males, and heart size is inversely related to heart rate (Bell et al. 1968).

Some laboratory studies, however, have shown that young adult males show greater heart rate reactivity than age-matched females in response to particular stressors (Frey and Siervogel 1983; Hastrup and Light 1984). Investigators have interpreted this apparent contradiction in light of evidence suggesting that the nature of the task and its gender-relevance may influence the direction of gender differences in heart rate responses. That is, if a task (e.g., speech delivery) is perceived to employ stereotypically female characteristics (e.g., empathy and submissiveness), young females show greater reactivity compared with males. On the other hand, if a challenge is perceived as one on which males typically excel (e.g., mental arithmetic), young males have been found to show greater heart rate increases compared with females (Girdler et al. 1990; Stoney et al. 1988). These data, however, are preliminary and remain to be substantiated by subsequent investigations.

Race and age effects on heart rate.   Most studies, whether epidemiologic or laboratory, indicate that young adult blacks generally show lower resting heart rates compared with their white counterparts, and that blacks show smaller stress-induced increases in heart rate relative to whites (N. B. Anderson et al. 1988a, 1988b; Falkner and Kushner 1989; Fredrikson 1986; Light and Sherwood 1989; Light et al. 1987; McAdoo et al. 1990; Myers et al. 1989; Tischenkel et al. 1989). With age, however, race differences in heart rate appear to diminish (Evans County studies, unpublished data cited in Persky et al. 1979; Persky et al. 1979). To date, no published studies exist that specifically investigate gender and race effects on stress-induced heart rate reactivity in the elderly.

Age Effects on Blood Pressure

Blood pressure, the strength with which blood moves through the arteries and blood vessels (Hassett 1978), is measured in units of millimeters of mercury. Systolic blood pressure is considered the peak arterial pressure produced when blood exits from the heart as it contracts. It is represented as the numerator of the ratio when systolic and diastolic blood pressures are expressed as a ratio. Diastolic pressure, the denominator in the pressure ratio, represents the force of blood flow present as the heart relaxes following contraction.

Numerous epidemiologic studies indicate that in most industrialized nations, resting systolic and diastolic blood pressures increase substantially with age (Epstein and Eckoff 1967; Whelton 1985). This increase in blood pressure, however, is not consistently seen among individuals in nonindustrialized societies.

With respect to stress-induced increases in blood pressure, a number of investigations have demonstrated that older individuals show greater stress-induced blood pressure reactivity relative to younger individuals. These results have been observed in studies using pharmacologic challenges, as well as across a variety of behavioral and cognitive challenges (Barnes et al. 1982; Faucheux et al. 1983; Garwood et al. 1982; Gintner et al. 1986; Matthews and Stoney 1988; Palmer et al. 1978; Powell et al. 1981; Wagner and Horvath 1985).

Investigators believe the augmented blood pressure responses seen in elderly relative to younger individuals are mediated by age-related cardiovascular changes including increases in total peripheral resistance, stroke volume, arterial rigidity, and left ventricular wall thickness, along with decreases in baroreceptor and beta-adrenergic sensitivity (Frey and Hoffler 1988; Gribbin et al. 1971; Pfeifer et al. 1983; Shimada et al. 1985). Consequently, diminished cardiac responsivity and increased vascular activity characterizes cardiovascular responses among older relative to younger individuals (Faucheux et al. 1983; Garwood et al. 1982; Gintner et al. 1986; Palmer et al. 1978; Pan et al. 1986; Powell et al. 1981; van Brummelen et al. 1981; Wagner and Horvath 1985).

Gender and age effects on blood pressure. Epidemiologic studies indicate that prior to the age of 50, resting systolic and diastolic blood pressures in males is higher than that in females (Forsman and Lindblad 1983; Frankenhaeuser et al. 1976; Jorgensen and Houston 1981; Liberson and Liberson 1975). After age 60 and older, however, females show higher resting blood pressures compared with males (Roberts and Rowland 1981).

With age and changes in reproductive hormone status, studies suggest that menopausal and postmenopausal women show greater reactivity to stressors compared with premenopausal women (Saab et al. 1989). These data are consistent with the epidemiologic data indicating an increased prevalence of cardiovascular disease in menopausal and postmenopausal women relative to premenopausal women (Kannel et al. 1976).

With regard to gender differences in reactivity, most laboratory studies show that young adult white males show larger stress-induced systolic blood pressure responses compared with age-matched females (Hastrup and Light 1984; Kannel et al. 1976; Matthews and Stoney 1988; McAdoo et al. 1990; Saab 1989; Stoney et al. 1988). However, as with the findings on gender and heart rate reactivity, gender differences in stress-induced blood pressure responses appear to be influenced by the gender-relevance of the stressor (for a review, see Saab 1989). Saab et al. (1989), for example, observed that a speech task requiring stereotypic female attributes elicited the greatest blood pressure reactivity among postmenopausal versus premenopausal women. On the other hand, no gender differences were observed in response to a number of stressors considered to be gender neutral or to have less personal relevance for females. These tasks included the cold pressor task, the Type A Stressful Interview, orthostatic stress, lower body negative pressure, mental arithmetic, and mirror image tracing

(Frey and Hoffler 1988; Girdler et al. 1990; Goldstein and Shapiro 1990; Tischenkel et al. 1989).

Race and age effects on blood pressure. Research has established that up to the age of 74, blacks show higher resting blood pressures compared with whites. Among individuals age 75 and older, however, whites show higher blood pressure compared with blacks (Roberts and Rowland 1981). Within genders, black women show a greater prevalence of elevated resting blood pressure relative to white women than black males do relative to white males (Roberts and Rowland 1981).

Studies on stress-induced blood pressure responses generally indicate that young and middle-age blacks show greater blood pressure reactivity compared with age-matched whites in response to a variety of stressors (N. B. Anderson et al. 1988a, 1989a; Durel et al. 1989; Light and Sherwood 1989; Light et al. 1987; McAdoo et al. 1990; McNeilly and Zeichner 1989; Tischenkel et al. 1989). A few studies, however, have not substantiated these findings (N. B. Anderson et al. 1988b; Falkner and Kushner 1989; Fredrikson 1986).

Interestingly, similar to the findings among older compared with younger individuals, studies suggest that the blood pressure elevations in blacks may be predominantly mediated by vascular mechanisms (vasoconstriction and peripheral resistance) rather than cardiac factors (heart rate and cardiac output), whereas the reverse may be true for whites (N. B. Anderson et al. 1988a, 1988b, 1989a, 1989b; Fredrikson 1986; Light and Sherwood 1989; Trieber et al. 1990). Again, however, not all studies support these findings (Light and Sherwood 1989; Parmer et al. 1990). Consequently, some investigators purport that individual rather than race differences are more important in determining cardiovascular responses to stress.

As of this writing, no published studies have specifically investigated the interactive effects of age, race, and gender on stress-induced blood pressure reactivity. Preliminary results from studies in our laboratory, however, suggest there are interactive effects of task, age, race, and gender on blood pressure reactivity. These findings have been presented at several national meetings and are soon to be submitted for publication.

Age Effects on Electrodermal Activity

Galvanic skin response, currently referred to as electrodermal activity, is a measure of the electrical activity of the skin. Briefly, electrodermal activity is quantified by measuring changes in skin conductance (the resistance encountered when passing a small electric current through the skin) or skin potential (bioelectric potential). These changes occur as a function of perspiration produced by the eccrine, or sweat, glands in response to a stressor (Hassett 1978; Stern et al. 1980). For a more complete description of electrodermal activity and its various methods of measurement, we recommend the text by Stern et al.

Several studies have shown that the number of active sweat glands and the amount of sweat produced per gland decreases with age (Juniper and Dykman 1967; MacKinnon 1954; Silver et al. 1964). These age-related changes are thought to account for the observed age differences in electrodermal activity. Investigations of a more methodological nature, however, indicate that procedural factors can influence the magnitude of the observed age differences in electrodermal activity. For example, larger age effects are obtained under experimental conditions of higher relative to lower epidermal resistance (Garwood et al. 1981). Furthermore, the anatomical site from which conductance is measured has been shown to influence the size of the obtained age effect (Capriotti et al. 1981).

Laboratory studies have shown that skin conductance levels at rest and in response to stress are reduced in older individuals. For example, in response to cognitive tasks such as mental arithmetic and a free-recall memory task, older individuals showed smaller increases in skin conductance compared with younger individuals (Furchtgott and Busemeyer

1979). Similarly, older individuals showed smaller skin conductance and skin potential responses compared with younger individuals in response to tones conditionally paired with electric shock (Shmavonian et al. 1965, 1968).

Gender and age effects on electrodermal activity. Investigations of gender effects on electrodermal activity have produced mixed results. These inconsistencies have been attributed to several factors. Females, for example, have been reported to show greater variability in electrodermal activity compared with males (Shmavonian et al. 1968). In addition, age and the type of stressor have been shown to influence both the direction and magnitude of gender effects on electrodermal activity. For instance, in response to a discrimination conditioning paradigm (pairing electric shock with tones), younger males showed greater skin conductance and skin potential responses relative to younger females (Shmavonian et al. 1968). With age, however, an opposite pattern emerged. That is, older women showed greater conditioned skin conductance and skin potential responses compared with older males. In contrast to these results, however, are those observed in response to the Valsalva maneuver where younger females showed larger skin conductance responses compared with males. Furthermore, younger females showed higher skin conductance responses compared with older females, whereas no age effect was seen for males (Eisdorfer et al. 1980).

Estrous also appears to have an effect on skin conductance levels in response to stimuli. Results from one study suggested premenopausal women showed lower resting skin conductance levels during the luteal phase and increases in skin conductance responses during the ovulatory phase in response to tones, time estimation, and a reaction time task. It was determined that 13% of the variation in skin conductance level was associated with the menstrual phase (Little and Zahn 1974).

Race and age effects on electrodermal activity. As of this writing, there are no published investigations of race effects on electrodermal activity in the elderly. Most studies of race differences in electrodermal activity among young adults, however, indicate that blacks show higher resting levels of skin resistance and lower conductance compared with whites. At present, these differences do not appear to be due to race differences in numbers of active sweat glands in black and white adults (Johnson and Landon 1965).

In contrast to the observed race differences in resting levels of skin resistance and conductance, no such differences have been observed among young adult blacks and whites in response to stress (Fisher and Kotses 1973; Johnson and Corah 1962; Johnson and Landon 1965; Juniper and Dykman 1967; Lieblich et al. 1973). These stressors, however, have largely consisted of auditory stimuli such as tones or bursts of white noise; the generalizability of these results to other stressors, therefore, is somewhat limited.

Age Effects on Catecholamine Responses

Catecholamines—norepinephrine, epinephrine, and dopamine—are neurotransmitters that are synthesized and stored in the neurons of the brain, ANS, and adrenal medulla. They are released in response to stress and exert excitatory effects on virtually all vital effector organs. Catecholamines can be measured in urine or in blood plasma. Urinary samples provide useful information regarding responses to stress over time but are not considered informative for measuring acute responses to stress. Plasma samples, on the other hand, are useful measures of acute stress responsivity, because blood levels of norepinephrine are known to correlate with sympathetic nerve activity.

A variety of techniques are available for the assay of catecholamines. Among them include high-performance liquid chromatography; radioenzymatic methods such as fluorometric, catechol-*O*-methyltransferase, and phenylethanolamine-*N*-methyltransferase assays; and gas chromatography. One of the most common methods used for catecholamine assay in many laboratories is high-performance liquid chromatography.

Readers should be aware that the collection, handling, and assay of plasma samples for catecholamine analysis is wrought with potential pitfalls too numerous to mention here. Hence, the informed investigator would do well to refer to such excellent sources as Ziegler (1989) to become apprised of optimal collection and assay strategies.

A large body of literature suggests that resting levels of plasma norepinephrine increase with age among normotensive individuals (Palmer et al. 1978; Ziegler et al. 1978). This increase is thought to be due to increased norepinephrine spillover rate or reduced norepinephrine clearance.

In response to a variety of stressors, older individuals have shown greater increases in plasma catecholamines relative to younger individuals. These stressors have included cognitive tasks such as memory recall and mental arithmetic, and physical stressors such as orthostatic stress, isometric exercise, and the cold pressor test (hand immersion in ice water) (Barnes et al. 1982; Palmer et al. 1978). In addition, compared with younger individuals, older persons have been shown to take longer to return to baseline levels of catecholamines following termination of the stressor (Lipsitz 1989).

Gender, race, and age effects on catecholamines. As of this writing, there are no published studies on gender and race differences in catecholamine responsivity in the elderly. Results from studies among younger individuals, however, suggest that males generally show greater urinary excretion of epinephrine than females in response to acute and chronic stress. Other studies of plasma catecholamine responses to stressors have failed to find significant differences between females and males in plasma catecholamines (for a review, see Saab 1989). Similarly, one study conducted with younger black and white adults yielded no significant race differences in norepinephrine and epinephrine (Tischenkel et al. 1989). Preliminary data from our laboratory and epidemiologic studies indicate, however, that healthy younger blacks show higher levels of baseline and stress-induced plasma catecholamines compared with their age-matched white counterparts. Studies of race differences in urinary dopamine have suggested that relative to whites, blacks have lower basal levels of urinary dopamine and beta-hydroxylase, a dopamine precursor (Berenson et al. 1979). Other studies have shown that blacks produce a blunted release of dopamine, a natriuretic agent, in response to a salt load (for a review, see Eisner 1990). Urinary dopamine excretion has also been shown to decrease with age among hypertensive individuals (for a review, see Zemel and Sowers 1988). These decreased levels of urinary dopamine among blacks and the elderly have been thought to be related to the earlier onset of hypertension among blacks and to the higher hypertension prevalence rates among blacks and the elderly.

Age Effects on Alpha-Adrenergic and Beta-Adrenergic Activity

ANS arousal is expressed by two patterns of adrenergic activity, referred to as the beta-adrenergic and alpha-adrenergic response patterns. These patterns of ANS responsivity have been studied primarily through the use of pharmacologic agonists and antagonists. The beta-adrenergic reactivity pattern is characterized by increases in heart rate, cardiac output, stroke volume, blood pressure, epinephrine, and norepinephrine and by a decrease in total peripheral resistance. In contrast to the beta-adrenergic pattern, the alpha-adrenergic pattern is associated with decreases in heart rate and cardiac output and increases in vasoconstriction, total peripheral resistance, and norepinephrine.

Beta-adrenergic activity has been studied extensively in the elderly. These studies have consistently demonstrated that, in both humans and animals, beta-adrenoceptor-mediated sensitivity to both agonists and antagonists decreases with age

(Bertel et al. 1980; Buhler 1983; Dillon et al. 1980; Fleisch 1980; Lakatta and Yin 1982; van Brummelen et al. 1981; Vestal et al. 1979). This decreased beta-adrenergic activity results in blunted stressor-induced heart rate, cardiac output, and vasodilatory responses and greater blood pressure increases in older compared with younger individuals (Garwood et al. 1982; Palmer et al. 1978; Pan et al. 1986; Powell et al. 1981; van Brummelen et al. 1981).

In contrast to the age-related reductions in beta-adrenergic sensitivity, evidence suggests that alpha$_1$- and alpha$_2$-adrenergic activity may not be attenuated in the elderly. For example, in response to the cold pressor task and ambient cold, stressors that elicit predominantly alpha$_1$-adrenergically mediated vasoconstriction, older individuals show greater increases in total peripheral resistance, plasma norepinephrine, and blood pressure compared with younger individuals (Palmer et al. 1978; Wagner and Horvath 1985). Other studies that have employed the pharmacologic challenge, clonidine, an alpha$_2$-adrenergic agonist, suggest that alpha$_2$-adrenergically mediated vasoconstriction is preserved in the elderly (Pan et al. 1986). The current research on alpha-adrenergic activity in the elderly, however, is somewhat controversial, and conclusions regarding age-related changes at this time are premature.

Gender and age effects on adrenergic activity. To our knowledge, no published studies have specifically examined gender effects on adrenergic activity in the elderly. In several studies conducted in young adult females, however, results indicated that females showed diminished peripheral vascular adrenergic receptor sensitivity, suggesting decreased sensitivity or density of alpha-adrenergic receptors or both (Freedman et al. 1987).

Race and age effects on adrenergic activity. As of this writing, no published studies have directly examined race effects on adrenergic activity in the elderly. Among young adults, however, one study has examined race differences in response to beta-adrenergic antagonism, alone and combined with behavioral stress (Light and Sherwood 1989). The results indicated that blacks showed greater vascular and cardiac reactivity to the beta-adrenergic antagonism. Another group of investigators (Parmer et al. 1990) used phentolamine, an alpha-adrenergic agonist, combined with stress to examine race differences in alpha-adrenergic activity. Their results yielded no significant race differences in cardiovascular responses to challenge.

Conceptual and Methodological Issues in Reactivity and Aging Research

Cohort, Period, and Time Effects

One of the most important considerations in aging research is differentiating between the effects of chronological age versus cohort and period effects. In certain fields of study, such as sociology, these factors frequently constitute the focus of study. In other areas of research, especially those that are more physiological, cohort and period effects are often neglected. These effects, however, can and do exert strong influences on physical, psychological, and behavioral responses. Therefore, distinguishing between age, period, and cohort effects in designing and interpreting gerontologic research clearly warrants attention.

Cohort effects reflect the influence of historical events that certain age groups may have experienced. These events may influence an elderly individual's responses to stress in the laboratory or in the natural environment. As such, observed age differences in physiological responses may be more a reflection of exposure to particular historical events rather than age effects per se. For example, age differences in physiological and psychological responses may be observed among older and younger Jewish individuals viewing films of Holocaust events. Differences in responses between the age groups, however, are likely not solely due to biological age effects, but to the fact that older and younger cohorts lived through different histori-cal events (e.g., pre- and post-World War II). Age group differ-ences in responses to certain stressors, therefore, could conceivably be a result of respective cohort experiences, rather than biological aging alone.

Period, or time of measurement, effects reflect the influ-ence of the present environment (Nesselroade and Labouvie 1985). For instance, in times of economic hardship, age differ-ences may be observed in attitudes concerning taxation aimed at increasing Social Security payments to the elderly. Older persons, for example, might favor taxation whereas younger individuals might hold the opposite view. This age difference in attitudes may influence how older and younger individuals respond to the same stimulus (in this case, an economic stress-or)—that of taxation to augment Social Security payments. Therefore, observed age differences may be a function of cur-rent period or time events rather than reflecting true biological age differences.

Health Status and Biological Factors

The effects of health and biological factors on physiological responses to stress present a particular challenge to geron-tologic investigators. That challenge is differentiating the effects of normal healthy aging from those of pathological changes that frequently accompany aging. The presence of disease, which is so frequently a part of the aging process, often confounds attempts to determine the effects of "nor-mal" aging.

Conceptual and methodological implications. The impli-cations of differentiating between healthy and pathological aging in stress-reactivity research are both conceptual and methodological. If illness is conceptualized as an intrinsic part of the aging process, theoretically, then the investigator would include all eligible subjects without regard to their medical status. Although this approach does not enable one to differentiate the effects of disease from the normal healthy aging process, it does allow the results to be extended to a more general population. On the other hand, if illness is viewed as distinct from aging and the effects of healthy aging per se are of interest, an approach consistent with this perspective is to screen and exclude all subjects for illnesses that may confound results. Although this strategy may allow the investigator to identify more directly mechanisms underlying normal healthy aging, this method is likely to result in a subject sample of biologically elite individuals who are not representative of the general population. For a more in-depth discussion of these issues, the reader is referred elsewhere (Rowe and Kahn 1987).

A third and most recommended approach combines the first two and allows the researcher to maximize both the interpretability and generalizability of the design. This method is to collect data on all subjects, healthy and diseased, and to analyze both the unscreened full sample and the screened subsample(s). Further analyses would then allow a more direct examination differentiating the effects of disease versus aging per se on the response system under investigation.

Health and fitness.   The prevalence of most major diseases—including cardiovascular diseases, hypertension, cancer, and diabetes—increases substantially with age. Irrespective of age, these diseases are more prevalent in blacks across the life span and are especially prevalent in black elderly persons up to age 75 (Jackson and Perry 1989; Report of the Secretary 1986). Each of these major diseases has been associated with stress-induced ANS dysregulation, and both the pathological processes and the medications used to treat them can influence physiological responses to stress. For example, studies have shown that blacks, individuals who have high resting blood pressure, borderline hypertensive persons, and individuals with established hypertension show greater cardiovascular and neuroendocrine reactivity to laboratory stressors (Fredrikson et al. 1982; Hollenberg et al. 1981; Light and Sherwood 1989;

Steptoe et al. 1984). In addition, whites with a parental history of hypertension show greater cardiovascular responses compared with the offspring of normotensive persons (Ditto 1986; Jorgensen and Houston 1981; Manuck and Proietti 1982). Consequently, we might expect these individuals to show greater responsivity in our stress research laboratories and clinic settings.

A number of investigations conducted with young adults have demonstrated that individuals at high levels of physical condition show attenuated cardiovascular and neuroendocrine reactivity to stressors relative to individuals at lower levels of physical condition (Blumenthal and McCubbin 1987; Dimsdale et al. 1986; Norris et al. 1990; Oleshansky et al. 1990).

Preliminary studies have been conducted in the elderly suggesting that older individuals who are physically fit may also show attenuated cardiovascular reactivity and augmented norepinephrine responsivity to stressors relative to their less-fit age-matched counterparts (Poehlman and Danforth 1991). The reasons for this discrepancy among response modalities may become apparent in our discussion of studies on stress reactivity later in this section.

Medications.   Medications that many elderly individuals are likely to take are also known to influence physiological responsivity. For example, beta-blockers have been shown to reduce heart rate and increase peripheral vascular responses to stress, especially in blacks and the elderly (e.g., see Light and Sherwood 1989).

Finally, the influence of exogenous estrogen on stress reactivity remains controversial. Findings from studies of stress reactivity in women taking estrogen in the form of hormone replacement therapy or oral contraceptives are mixed. Results from these studies have shown that in some cases oral contraceptives may attenuate cardiovascular reactivity to stress (Marinari et al. 1976; Neus and von Eiff 1985) and in others to augment (Emmons and Weidner 1988) stress-induced reactivity.

Hormonal factors. Studies have shown that age-related changes in reproductive hormones among females may affect physiological responses to stress. These studies have shown that menopausal and postmenopausal women not taking contraceptive or replacement estrogen show greater reactivity to stressors compared with premenopausal women (Saab et al. 1989). Findings such as these have been interpreted in light of evidence suggesting that estrogen may protect against cardiovascular disease, possibly through mechanisms of lipid metabolism (Barrett-Connor and Bush 1988).

Health behaviors. Cigarette smoking, caffeine, and dietary sodium intake have been shown to increase reactivity to stress (Ambrosioni et al. 1982; Luft et al. 1977; Pomerleau and Pomerleau 1987). To the degree that these behaviors differ across age, race, and gender groupings, they may explain group differences in physiological responding. For example, smoking rates are significantly higher in blacks (Novotny et al. 1988), in males (Waldron 1986), and in persons with lower socioeconomic status (Novotny et al. 1988). Also, although dietary sodium intake may not be higher in blacks (Grim et al. 1980), its effects on blood pressure are greater (Luft et al. 1977). Lastly, studies suggest that sodium excretion is reduced in the elderly relative to younger individuals (Luft et al. 1979; Weinberger and Fineberg 1991). Conceivably, if endogenous sodium levels are higher in the elderly, this could contribute to their augmented resting and stress-induced blood pressures, because sodium is known to stimulate the release of norepinephrine and augment its vasoconstrictive effects.

Applications of Stress-Reactivity Research in Clinical Settings

Within recent years there has been a growing awareness among clinicians, researchers, and laypersons that certain physical and psychological syndromes may be precipitated or exacerbated by exposure to stressors. These psychological or psychiatric conditions include anxiety (including posttraumatic stress disorder) and affective, personality, psychosexual, and thought disorders (for a review, see Ray et al. 1983). Physical diseases that have been linked to stress responsivity include hypertension and cardiovascular diseases (Blanchard et al. 1988; Krantz et al. 1986; Krantz and Manuck 1984; Matthews et al. 1986; Schneiderman et al. 1989), diabetes (Surwit and Feinglos 1983), headaches (Blanchard and Andrasik 1985), neuromuscular problems (Baker 1979; Basmajian et al. 1977; DeBacher 1979), and chronic pain (Keefe and Hoelscher 1987; Keefe et al. 1981).

Epidemiologic research indicates that the prevalence rates for many of these disorders substantially increase with increasing age (Haan et al. 1987; Hing et al. 1983; Markides 1989; Report of the Secretary 1986). Because stress has been shown to precipitate or exacerbate symptoms in these diseases, some investigators have hypothesized that stress-induced physiological responses may contribute to the augmented prevalence rates of these stress-related diseases among the elderly.

In clinical settings, treatment of stress-related disorders has included interventions such as biofeedback, autogenic training, relaxation training, hypnosis, guided imagery, stress management, and systematic desensitization. These interventions, which are largely based on theories of classical and operant conditioning, have helped individuals cope with or alleviate their stress-related disorders. For more comprehensive discussions of the assessment and treatment of stress-related disorders, we recommend two excellent texts (Golberger and Breznitz 1982; Woolfolk and Lehrer 1984).

Summary, Discussion, and Future Directions

We presented the theoretical basis for stress-reactivity research and a summary of selected research on age differences in physiological responses to stress. When available, we included data on the interactive effects of race, gender, and age. Presentation of these findings was followed by a discussion of certain conceptual and methodological issues relative to gerontologic research. Lastly, various applications of stress-reactivity research in clinical settings for the assessment and treatment of stress-related disorders were outlined.

In our presentation of the data on age differences in physiological responses to stress, it is strikingly apparent that although race and gender effects are currently under study in younger individuals, such investigations are distinctly lacking in elderly individuals. In light of findings demonstrating that responses to stress do indeed differ across race and gender in younger individuals, research on the interactive effects of these variables with age is clearly warranted.

Relatedly, in discussing these findings, we have made little mention of the psychosocial and environmental factors that may modulate responses to stress. Most gerontologic research, in fact, assumes that differences in physiological responses are the result of biological or genetic factors. Psychosocial and environmental factors may play important roles in modulating group differences in response to stress. Although it is beyond the scope of this chapter to provide an in-depth presentation of this topic, a more detailed discussion may be found elsewhere (N. B. Anderson and McNeilly 1991). Suffice it to say here that to the extent these modulating factors differ across age, race, and gender, they contribute to the observed group differences in physiological responses. To cite one among many possible examples, socioeconomic status is strongly associated with increasing age, black race, and female gender (Farley and Allen 1989; Longino et al. 1989). Because low socioeconomic status and exposure to stress have been linked to ANS dysregulation (elevated blood pressure and catecholamine levels), somatic symptoms, anxiety, and depression (Baum et al. 1983; Davidson et al. 1987; Fleming et al. 1987a, 1987b; Haan et al. 1987; Harburg et al. 1973; James and Kleinbaum 1976; Kessler and Neighbors 1986; Kessler et al. 1987, 1988), one implication for the clinical geriatrician or gerontologic researcher is that individuals at lower levels of socioeconomic status (particularly if they are elderly, black, or female) may likely exhibit augmented resting levels of ANS activity and exaggerated reactivity to stress. These differences in physiological responses, however, may be more likely a consequence of their exposure to the social and environmental stressors associated with lower socioeconomic status and less likely due to biological constitutional differences.

These findings along with others suggest that gerontologic researchers and geriatric clinicians must be sensitive to psychosocial and socioecologic factors that may influence or perhaps account for the magnitude and patterns of the observed stress responsivity. It is our belief that more research is needed that is aimed at determining the contextual basis for the frequent observations of age, gender, and race differences in stress reactivity. For an in-depth presentation and discussion of this contextual perspective, the reader is referred elsewhere (N. B. Anderson and McNeilly 1991). Research of this nature may facilitate our understanding of biological, psychological, behavioral, environmental, and sociocultural interactions on stressor-induced physiological responses in laboratory and clinical settings and may assist in identifying factors responsible for sociodemographic group differences in health morbidity and mortality.

References

Ambrosioni E, Costa FV, Borghi S, et al: Effects of moderate salt restriction on intralymphocytic sodium and pressor response to stress in borderline hypertension. Hypertension 4:789–794, 1982

Anderson DE, Kearns WD, Better WE: Progressive hypertension in dogs by avoidance conditioning and saline infusion. Hypertension 5:286–291, 1983

Anderson NB, McNeilly M: Age, gender, and ethnicity as variables in psychophysiological assessment: sociodemographics in context. Psychological Assessment: J Consult Clin Psychol 3:376–384, 1991

Anderson NB, Lane JD, Williams RB Jr, et al: Racial differences in blood pressure and forearm vascular responses to the cold face stimulus. Psychosom Med 50:57–63, 1988a

Anderson NB, Lane JD, Monou H, et al: Racial differences in cardiovascular responses to mental arithmetic. Int J Psychophysiol 6:161–164, 1988b

Anderson NB, Lane JD, Taguchi F, et al: Patterns of cardiovascular responses to stress as a function of race and parental hypertension in men. Health Psychol 8:525–540, 1989a

Anderson NB, Lane JD, Taguchi F, et al: Race parental history of hypertension, and patterns of cardiovascular reactivity in women. Psychophysiology 26:39–47, 1989b

Baker MP: Biofeedback in specific muscle retraining, in Biofeedback—Principles and Practice for Clinicians. Edited by Basmajian JV. Baltimore, MD, Williams & Wilkins, 1979, pp 81–91

Barnes RF, Raskind M, Gumbrecht G, et al: The effects of age on the plasma catecholamine response to mental stress in man. J Clin Endocrinol Metab 54:64–69, 1982

Barnett PH, Hines KA, Schirger A, et al: Blood pressure and vascular reactivity to the cold pressor test. JAMA 183:845–848, 1963

Barrett-Connor E, Bush TL: Estrogen replacement and coronary heart disease. Cardiovasc Clin 19:159–172, 1988

Basmajian JV, Regenos E, Baker M: Rehabilitating stroke patients with biofeedback. Geriatrics 32:85–88, 1977

Baum A, Gatchel RJ, Schaeffer MA: Emotional behavioral, and physiological effects of chronic stress at Three Mile Island. J Consult Clin Psychol 51:565–572, 1983

Bell GH, Davidson JN, Scarborough H (eds): Textbook of Physiology and Biochemistry. London, Livingstone, 1968

Berenson G, Voors A, Webber L, et al: Racial differences in parameters associated with blood pressure levels in children: the Bogalusa Heart Study. Metabolism 28:1218–1228, 1979

Bertel O, Buhler FR, Kiowski W, et al: Decreased beta-adrenoreceptor responsiveness as related to age, blood pressure, and plasma catecholamines in patients with essential hypertension. Hypertension 2:130–138, 1980

Blanchard EB, Andrasik F (eds): Management of Chronic Headaches: A Psychological Approach. New York, Pergamon, 1985

Blanchard EB, Martin JE, Dubbert PM (eds): Non-drug Treatments for Essential Hypertension. New York, Pergamon, 1988

Blumenthal JA, McCubbin JA: Physical exercise as stress management, in the Handbook of Psychology and Health, Vol 5:Stress. Edited by Baum A, Singer JE. Hillsdale, NJ, Lawrence Erlbaum Associates, 1987, pp 303–331

Borghi C, Costa FV, Boschi S, et al: Predictors of stable hypertension in young borderline subjects: a five-year follow-up study. J Cardiovasc Pharmacol 8:S138–141, 1986

Buhler FR: Age and cardiovascular response adaptation. Hypertension 5 (suppl 3):94–100, 1983

Cacioppo JT, Petty RE: Social Psychophysiology: A Sourcebook. New York, Guilford, 1983

Capriotti R, Garwood M, Engel BT: Skin potential level: age and recording site interactions. J Gerontol 36:40–43, 1981

Coles MG, Donchin E, Porges SW (eds): Psychophysiology: Systems, Processes, and Applications. New York, Guilford, 1986

Collins A, Frankenhaeuser M: Stress response in male and female engineering students. Journal of Human Stress 4:43–48, 1978

Davidson LM, Fleming R, Baum A: Chronic stress, catecholamines, and sleep disturbance at Three Mile Island. Journal of Human Stress 13:75–83, 1987

DeBacher G: Biofeedback in spasticity control, in Biofeedback—Principles and Practice for Clinicians. Edited by Basmajian JV. Baltimore, MD, Williams & Wilkins, 1979

Dillon N, Chung S, Kelly J, et al: Age and beta adrenoceptor-mediated function. Clin Pharmacol Ther 27:769–772, 1980

Dimsdale JE, Alpert BS, Schneiderman N: Exercise as a modulator of cardiovascular reactivity, in the Handbook of Stress Reactivity and Cardiovascular Disease. Edited by Matthews K, Weiss SM, Detre T, et al. New York, Wiley, 1986, pp 365–384

Ditto B: Parental history of essential hypertension, active coping, and cardiovascular reactivity. Psychophysiology 23:62–70, 1986

Durel LA, Carver CS, Spitzer SB, et al: Associations of blood pressure with self-report measures of anger and hostility among black and white men and women. Health Psychol 8:557–575, 1989

Eich RH, Jacobensen EC: Vascular reactivity in medical students followed for 10 years. Journal of Chronic Diseases 20:583–592, 1967

Eisdorfer C, Doerr HO, Follette W: Electrodermal reactivity: an analysis by age and sex. Journal of Human Stress 6:39–42, 1980

Eisner GM: Hypertension: Racial differences. Am J Kidney Dis 16:35–40, 1990

Emmons KM, Weidner G: The effects of cognitive and physical stress on cardiovascular reactivity among smokers and oral contraceptive users. Psychophysiology 25:166–171, 1988

Epstein FH, Eckoff RD: The epidemiology of high blood pressure: geographic distribution and etiological factors, in The Epidemiology of Hypertension. Edited by Stammler J, Pullman R. New York, Grune & Stratton, 1967, pp 155–166

Falkner B, Kushner H: Race differences in stress-induced reactivity in young adults. Health Psychol 8:613–627, 1989

Farley R, Allen WR: The Color Line and the Quality of Life in America. New York, Oxford University Press, 1989

Faucheux BA, Dupuis C, Baulon A, et al: Heart rate reactivity during minor mental stress in men in their 50s and 70s. Gerontology 29:149–160, 1983

Finch CE: Neuroendocrine and autonomic aspects of aging, in The Handbook of the Biology of Aging. Edited by Finch CE, Hayflick L. New York, Van Nostrand Reinhold, 1977, pp 262–280

Fisher LE, Kotses H: Race relations and experimenter race effect in galvanic skin response. Psychophysiology 10:578–582, 1973

Fleg JL, Tzankoff SP, Lakatta EG: Age-related augmentation of plasma catecholamines during dynamic exercise in healthy males. J Appl Physiol 59:1033–1039, 1985

Fleisch JH: Age-related changes in the sensitivity of blood vessels to drugs. Pharmacol Ther 8:477–487, 1980

Fleming I, Baum A, Davidson LM, et al: Chronic stress as a factor in psychologic reactivity to challenge. Health Psychol 6:221–238, 1987a

Fleming I, Baum A, Weiss L: Social density and perceived control as mediators of crowding stress in high-density residential neighborhoods. J Pers Soc Psychol 52:899–906, 1987b

Folkow B: Psychosocial and central nervous influences in primary hypertension. Circulation 76 (Supp 1):110–119, 1987

Folkow B, Grimby G, Thulesius O: Adaptive structural changes of the vascular walls in hypertension and their relation to the control of the peripheral resistance. Acta Physiol Scand 44:255–272, 1958

Forsman L, Lindblad LE: Effect of mental stress on baroreceptor-mediated changes in blood pressure and heart rate and on plasma catecholamines and subjective responses in healthy men and women. Psychosom Med 45:435–445, 1983

Frankenhaeuser M, Dunne E, Lundberg U: Sex differences in sympathetic-adrenal medullary reactions induced by different stressors. Psychopharmacology 47:1–5, 1976

Fredrikson M: Racial differences in reactivity to behavioral challenge in essential hypertension. J Hypertens 4:325–331, 1986

Fredrikson M, Dimberg U, Frisk-Hamber M, et al: Hemodynamic and electrodermal correlates of psychogenic stimuli in normotensive and hypertensive subjects. Biol Psychol 15:63–73, 1982

Freedman RR, Sabharwal SC, Desai N: Sex differences in peripheral vascular adrenergic receptors. Circ Res 61:581–585, 1987

Frey MA, Hoffler GW: Association of sex and age with responses to lower-body negative pressure. J Appl Physiol 65:1752–1756, 1988

Frey MA, Siervogel RM: Cardiovascular response to a mentally stressful stimulus. Jpn Heart J 24:315–323, 1983

Furchtgott E, Busemeyer JK: Heart rate and skin conductance during cognitive processes as a function of age. J Gerontol 34:183–190, 1979

Garwood M, Engel BT, Kusterer JP: Skin potential level: age and epidermal hydration effects. J Gerontol 36:7–13, 1981

Garwood M, Engel BT, Capriotti R: Autonomic nervous system function and aging: response specificity. Psychophysiology 19:378–385, 1982

Gintner GG, Hollandsworth JG, Intrieri RC: Age differences in cardiovascular reactivity under active coping conditions. Psychophysiology 23:113–120, 1986

Girdler SS, Turner JR, Sherwood A, et al: Gender differences in blood pressure control during a variety of behavioral stressors. Psychosom Med 52:571–591, 1990

Goldberger L, Breznitz S (eds): Handbook of Stress. New York, Free Press, 1982

Goldstein IB, Shapiro D: Cardiovascular response during postural change in the elderly. J Gerontol 45:M20–M25, 1990

Goldstraw PW, Warren DJ: The effect of age on the cardiovascular responses to isometric exercise: a test of autonomic function. Gerontology 31:54–58, 1985

Gribbin B, Pickering TG, Sleight P, et al: Effect of age and high blood pressure on baroreflex sensitivity in man. Circ Res 29:424–431, 1971

Grim C, Luft F, Miller J, et al: Racial differences in blood pressure in Evans County, Georgia: relationship to sodium and potassium intake and plasma renin activity. J Chronic Dis 33:87–94, 1980

Haan M, Kaplan GA, Camacho T: Poverty and health. Am J Epidemiol 125:989–998, 1987

Hallback M, Folkow B: Cardiovascular response to acute mental "stress" in spontaneously hypertensive rats. Acta Physiol Scand 90:684–693, 1974

Harburg E, Erfurt J, Hauenstein L, et al: Socioecological stress suppressed hostility, skin color, and black-white blood pressure: Detroit. J Chronic Dis 26:595–611, 1973

Harlan WR, Osborne RK, Graybiel A: Prognostic value of the cold pressor test and the basal blood pressure: based on an 18-year follow-up study. Am J Cardiol 13:683–687, 1964

Hassett J: A Primer of Psychophysiology. San Francisco, CA, WH Freeman, 1978

Hastrup JL, Light KC: Sex differences in cardiovascular stress responses: modulation as a function of menstrual cycle phases. J Psychosom Res 28:475–483, 1984

Henry JP, Cassel J: Psychosocial factors in essential hypertension: recent epidemiologic and animal experimental evidence. Am J Epidemiol 90:171–200, 1969

Henry JP, Stephens PM, Santisteban GA: A model of psychosocial hypertension showing reversibility and progression of complications. Circ Res 36:156–164, 1975

Hing E, Kovar MG, Rice DP: Vital and Health Statistics (Series 3, No 24): Sex differences in health and use of medical care in the United States, 1979 (DHHS Publ No PHS 83). Hyattsville, MD, National Center for Health Statistics, 1983

Hollenberg NK, Williams GH, Adams DF: Essential hypertension: abnormal renal vascular and endocrine responses to a mild psychological stimulus. Hypertension 3:11–17, 1981

Jackson JJ, Perry C: Physical health conditions of middle-aged and aged blacks, in Aging and Health: Perspectives on Gender, Race, Ethnicity, and Class. Edited by Markides KS. Beverly Hills, CA, Sage, 1989, pp 111–176

Jackson AS, Squires WG, Grimes G, et al: Predicting future resting hypertensives from exercise and blood pressure. Journal of Cardiac Rehabilitation 3:263–268, 1983

James SA, Kleinbaum DG: Socioecologic stress and hypertension-related mortality rates in North Carolina. Am J Public Health 66:354–358, 1976

Johnson LC, Corah NL: Racial differences in skin resistance. Science 139:766–767, 1962

Johnson LC, Landon M: Eccrine sweat gland activity and racial differences in resting skin conductance. Psychophysiology 1:322–329, 1965

Jorgensen RS, Houston BK: Family history of hypertension, gender, and cardiovascular reactivity and stereotypy during stress. J Behav Med 4:175–189, 1981

Jose AD: Effect of combined sympathetic and parasympathetic blockade on heart rate and cardiac function in men. Am J Cardiol 18:476–478, 1966

Juniper K, Dykman RA: Skin resistance, sweat gland counts, salivary flow, and gastric secretion: Age, race and sex differences and intercorrelations. Psychophysiology 4:216–222, 1967

Kannel WB, Hjortland MC, McNamara PM, et al: Menopause and risk of cardiovascular disease: the Framingham Study. Ann Intern Med 85:446–452, 1976

Keefe FJ, Hoelscher T: Biofeedback in the management of chronic pain syndromes: Biofeedback Society of America task force report, in Biofeedback: Studies in Clinical Efficacy. Edited by Hatch JP, Fisher JG, Rugh JD. New York, Plenum, 1987, pp 211–253

Keefe FJ, Schapira B, Brown C, et al: EMG-assisted relaxation training in the management of chronic low back pain. American Journal of Clinical Biofeedback 4:93–103, 1981

Kessler RC, Neighbors HW: A new perspective on the relationship among race, social class, and psychological distress. J Health Soc Behav 27:107–115, 1986

Kessler RC, Turner JB, House JS: Intervening processes in the relationship between unemployment and health. Psychol Med 17:949–961, 1987

Kohn RR: Heart and cardiovascular system, in The Handbook of the Biology of Aging. Edited by Finch CE, Hayflick L. New York, Van Nostrand Reinhold, 1977, pp 281–317

Krantz DS, Manuck SB, Wing RR: Psychological stressors and task variables as elicitors of reactivity, in Handbook of Stress Reactivity and Cardiovascular Disease. Edited by Matthews KA, Weiss SM, Detre T, et al. New York, Wiley, 1986, pp 85–107

Lakatta EG, Yin FCP: Myocardial aging: functional alterations and related cellular mechanisms. Am J Physiol 242:H927–H941, 1982

Liberson CW, Liberson WT: Sex differences in autonomic responses to electric shock. Psychophysiology 12:182–186, 1975

Lieblich I, Kugelmass S, Ben-Shakhar G: Psychophysiological baselines as a function of race and origin. Psychophysiology 10:426–430, 1973

Light KC, Sherwood A: Race, borderline hypertension, and hemodynamic responses to behavioral stress before and after beta-adrenergic blockade. Health Psychol 8:577–595, 1989

Light KC, Obrist PA, Sherwood A, et al: Effects of race and marginally elevated blood pressure on cardiovascular responses to stress in young men. Hypertension 10:555–563, 1987

Lipsitz LA, Marks ER, Koestner J, et al: Reduced susceptibility to syncope during postural tilt in old age: is betabockade protective? Arch Intern Med 149:2709–2712, 1989

Little BC, Zahn TP: Changes in mood and autonomic functioning during the menstrual cycle. Psychophysiology 11:579–590, 1974

Longino CF Jr, Warheit GJ, Green JA: Class, aging, and health, in Aging and Health: Perspectives on Gender, Race, Ethnicity, and Class. Edited by Markides KS. Beverly Hills, CA, Sage, 1989, 79–109

Luft F, Grim C, Higgins J, et al: Differences in response to sodium administration in normotensive White and Black subjects. J Lab Clin Med 90:555–562, 1977

Luft F, Grim C, Fineberg N, et al: Effects of volume expansion and contraction in normotensive whites, blacks, and subjects of different ages. Circulation 59:643–650, 1979

Lundin S, Thoren P: Renal function and sympathetic activity during mental stress in normotensive and spontaneously hypertensive rats. Acta Physiol Scand 115:115–124, 1982

MacKinnon DCB: Variation with age in the number of active palmar digital sweat glands. J Neurol Neurosurg Psychiatry 17:124–126, 1954

Manuck SB, Proietti JM: Parental hypertension and cardiovascular response to cognitive and isometric challenge. Psychophysiology 19:481–489, 1982

Manuck SB, Kasprowicz AL, Muldoon MF: Behaviorally evoked cardiovascular reactivity potential associations. Ann Behav Med 12:17–29, 1990

Marinari KT, Leshner AI, Doyle MP: Menstrual cycle status and adrenocortical reactivity to psychological stress. Psychoneuroendocrinology 1:213–218, 1976

Markides KS (ed): Aging and Health: Perspectives on Gender, Race, Ethnicity, and Class. Beverly Hills, CA, Sage, 1989

Matthews KA, Stoney CM: Influences of sex and age on cardiovascular responses during stress. Psychosom Med 50:46–56, 1988

Matthews K, Weiss S, Detre T, et al (eds): Handbook of Stress Reactivity and Cardiovascular Disease. New York, Wiley, 1986

McAdoo WG, Weinberger MH, Miller JZ, et al: Race and gender influence hemodynamic responses to psychological and physical stimuli. J Hypertens 8:961–967, 1990

McNeilly M, Zeichner A: Neuropeptide and cardiovascular responses to intravenous catheterization in normotensive and hypertensive blacks and whites. Health Psychol 8:487–501, 1989

Menkes MS, Matthews KA, Krantz DS, et al: Cardiovascular reactivity to the cold pressor test as a predictor of hypertension. Hypertension 14:524–530, 1989

Myers HF, Shapiro D, McClure F, et al: Impact of caffeine and psychological stress on blood pressure in black and white men. Health Psychol 8:597–612, 1989

Nesselroade JR, Labouvie EW: Experimental design in research on aging, in The Handbook of The Psychology of Aging, 2nd Edition. Edited by Birren JE, Schaie KW. New York, Van Nostrand Reinhold, 1985, pp 35–60

Neus H, von Eiff AW: Selected topics in the methodology of stress testing: time course, gender, and adaptation, in Clinical and Methodological Issues in Cardiovascular Psychophysiology. Edited by Steptoe A, Ruddel H, Neus H. Berlin, Germany, Springer-Verlag, 1985, pp 78–92

Norris R, Carroll D, Cochrane R: The effects of aerobic and anaerobic training on fitness, blood pressure, and psychological stress and well-being. J Psychosom Res 34:367–375, 1990

Novotny TE, Warner KE, Kendrick JS, et al: Smoking by blacks and whites: socioeconomic and demographic differences. Am J Public Health 9:1187–1189, 1988

Obrist PA: Cardiovascular Psychophysiology: A Perspective. New York, Plenum, 1981

Oleshansky MA, Zoltick JM, Herman RH, et al: The influence of fitness on neuroendocrine responses to exhaustive treadmill exercise. Eur J Appl Physiol 59:405–410, 1990

Palmer GJ, Ziegler MG, Lake CR: Response of norepinephrine and blood pressure to stress increases with age. J Gerontol 33:482–487, 1978

Pan HYM, Hoffman BB, Perske RA, et al: Decline in beta-adrenergic receptor-mediated vascular relaxation with aging in man. J Pharmacol Exp Ther 239:802–807, 1986

Parmer RJ, Cervenka JH, Stone RA, et al: Autonomic function in hypertension: are there racial differences? Circulation 81:1305–1311, 1990

Persky V, Dyer A, Stamler J, et al: Racial patterns of heart rate in an employed adult population. Am J Epidemiol 110:274–280, 1979

Pfeifer MA, Weinberg CR, Cook D, et al: Differential changes of autonomic nervous system function with age in men. Am J Med 75:249–258, 1983

Pickering G, Gerin W: Area review: blood pressure reactivity: cardiovascular reactivity in the laboratory and the role of behavioral factors in hypertension: a critical review. Ann Behav Med 12:3–16, 1990

Poehlman ET, Danforth E: Endurance training increases metabolic rate and norepinephrine appearance in older individuals. Program abstracts, 44th Annual Scientific Meeting of the Gerontological Society of America, 1991

Pomerleau CS, Pomerleau OF: The effects of psychological stressor on cigarette smoking and subsequent behavioral and physiological responses. Psychophysiology 24:278–285, 1987

Powell DA, Milligan WL, Furchtgott E: Peripheral autonomic changes accompanying learning and reaction time performance in older people. J Gerontol 36:57–65, 1981

Ray WJ, Cole HW, Raczynski JM: Psychophysiological assessment, in The Clinical Psychology Handbook. Edited by Hersen M, Kazdin AE, Bellack AS. New York, Pergamon, 1983, pp 465–490

Report of the Secretary: Task Force on Black and Minority Health, Vol 4: Cardiovascular and Cerebrovascular Disease, Part I. Washington, DC, U.S. Department of Health and Human Services, 1986

Roberts J, Rowland M: Vital and Health Statistics (Series 11, No 221): Hypertension in adults 25-74 years of age: United States, 1971–75 (DHEW Publ No PHS 81). Washington, DC, U.S. Government Printing Office, 1981

Rowe JW, Kahn RL: Human aging: usual and successful. Science 237:143–149, 1987

Saab PG: Cardiovascular and neuroendocrine responses to challenge in males and females, in The Handbook of Research Methods in Cardiovascular Behavioral Medicine. Edited by Schneiderman N, Weiss SM, Kaufmann PG. New York, Plenum, 1989, pp 453–481

Saab PG, Matthews KA, Stoney CM, et al: Premenopausal and postmenopausal women differ in their cardiovascular and neuroendocrine responses to behavioral stressors. Psychophysiology 26:270–280, 1989

Sato I, Hasegawa Y, Takahashi N, et al: Age related changes of cardiac control function in man: with special reference to heart rate control at rest and during exercise. J Gerontol 36:564–572, 1981

Schneiderman N, Weiss SM, Kaufmann PG (eds): Handbook of Research Methods in Cardiovascular Behavioral Medicine. New York, Plenum, 1989

Shimada K, Kitazumi T, Sadakane N, et al: Age-related changes of baroreflex function, plasma norepinephrine, and blood pressure. Hypertension 7:113–117, 1985

Shmavonian BM, Yarmat AJ, Cohen SI: Relationships between the autonomic nervous system and central nervous system in age differences in behavior, in Behavior, Aging and the Nervous System. Edited by Welford AT, Birren JE. Springfield, IL, Charles C Thomas, 1965, pp 235–238

Shmavonian BM, Miller LH, Cohen SI: Differences among age and sex groups in electrodermal conditioning. Psychophysiology 5:119–131, 1968

Silver A, Montagna W, Karacan I: Age and sex differences in spontaneous adrenergic and cholinergic human sweating. J Invest Dermatol 43:255–265, 1964

Steptoe A, Melville D, Ross A: Behavioral response demands, cardiovascular reactivity and essential hypertension. Psychosom Med 46:33–48, 1984

Stern RM, Ray WJ, Davis CM (eds): Psychophysiological Recording. New York, Oxford University Press, 1980

Stoney CM, Matthews KA, McDonald RH, et al: Sex differences in lipid, lipoprotein, cardiovascular, and neuroendocrine responses to acute stress. Psychophysiology 25: 645–656, 1988

Surwit RS, Feinglos MN: The effects of relaxation on glucose tolerance in non-insulin-dependent diabetes mellitus. Diabetes Care 6:176–179, 1983

Tischenkel NJ, Saab PG, Schneiderman N, et al: Cardiovascular and neurohumoral responses to behavioral challenge as a function of race and sex. Health Psychol 8:503–524, 1989

Trieber FA, Musante L, Braden D, et al: Racial differences in hemodynamic responses to the cold face stimulus in children and adults. Psychosom Med 52:286–296, 1990

van Brummelen P, Buhler FR, Kiowski W, et al: Age-related decrease in cardiac and peripheral vascular responsiveness to isoprenaline: studies in normal subjects. Clin Sci 60:571–577, 1981

Vestal RE, Wood AJ, Shand DG: Reduced beta-adrenoceptor sensitivity in the elderly. Clin Pharmacol Ther 26:181–186, 1979

Wagner JA, Horvath SM: Cardiovascular reactions to cold exposures differ with age and gender. J Appl Physiol 58:185–192, 1985

Waldron I: The contribution of smoking to sex differences in mortality. Public Health Rep 101:163–173, 1986

Weinberger M, Fineberg N: Sodium and volume sensitivity of blood pressure: age and pressure change over time. Hypertension 18:67–71, 1991

Whelton PK: Blood pressure in adults and the elderly, in The Handbook of Hypertension, Vol 6: Epidemiology of Hypertension. Edited by Bulpitt CJ. New York, Elsevier Science, 1985

Wood DL, Sheps SG, Elveback LR, et al: Cold pressor test as a predictor of hypertension. Hypertension 6:301–306, 1984

Woolfolk RL, Lehrer PM (eds): Principles and Practice of Stress Management. New York, Guilford, 1984

Zemel MB, Sowers JR: Salt sensitivity and systemic hypertension in the elderly. Am J Cardiol 61:7H–12H, 1988

Ziegler MG: Catecholamine measurement in behavioral research, in The Handbook of Research Methods in Cardiovascular Behavioral Medicine. Edited by Schneiderman N, Weiss SM, Kaufmann PG. New York, Plenum, 1989, pp 167–183

Ziegler MG, Lake CR, Kopin IJ: Plasma noradrenaline increases with age. Nature 261:333–335, 1976

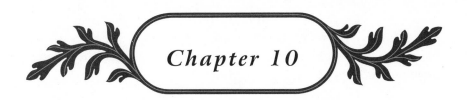

Chapter 10

Behavioral and Physiological Responses to Stress in Aging Animals

Mark J. Rosenthal, M.D.

I n this chapter, selected age-related changes in behavioral and hormonal responses to stress-ful situations in rodents are discussed. Mice and rats serve as useful models for the investigation of stress reactions with age. The neurophysiology and hormonal programming of these animals are well studied, and their life span is limited to 3 years. Varying severities of stressors can be inflicted on animals, and the behavioral and hormonal responses observed. In addition, stress responses are hormonally similar in rodents and humans.

To understand the effect of age on rodents' behavioral and hormonal responses to stress, it is first necessary to examine age-related changes in rodents that occur independently of stress. Therefore, in the first section of this chapter, changes in behaviors and endocrine functioning that occur with aging are described. The behaviors and hormonal responses in rodents that typically occur with stress are then reviewed. Finally, the interaction of stress and age on these behaviors and hormonal responses is described.

Changes in Motor Performance With Age

The capacity for movement, the sensorimotor skills entailed in making those movements that typically increase with stress, and vigor and vitality decline with age. Comparing rats ages 6, 12, 24, and 30 months, age-related declines were observed in the ability to localize stimuli and in hind-limb placing and stepping reactions (Marshall 1982). Limb reflexes were markedly slowed and tone reduced in rats 24 months and older. Old mice have difficulty climbing along a suspended rope (Miquel and Blasco 1976), climbing on a wire mesh, hanging from a horizontal wire (Wallace et al. 1980), and swimming in a tank of water (Marshall and Berrios 1979).

Yet, despite these decrements, in an unstressed situation, only selected activities decline with age. We (Rosenthal et al. 1989) and others (Janicke et al. 1983) reported no significant effects of age on basal or spontaneous activity. We did observe a nonsignificant trend toward greater rearing in the 3-month compared with 12- and 24-month Fischer rats. In mice, which rear far less frequently than rats, we saw no differences in home cage behavior between 10- and 27-month animals (Rosenthal and Morley 1989); others reported lower motor activity in 30-month but not in 24-month mice (Thurmond and Heishman 1984).

However, we did find a significant age-related difference in minimal stimulation of 27- versus 10-month C57Bl mice (Rosenthal et al. 1988) when placed for 30 minutes into an activity box, as monitored by disruption of a photo beam (see Table 10–1). Startle amplitude was diminished after white noise stimulation but not after electric shock in rats up to 30 months old (Krauter et al. 1981).

Changes in Neuroendocrine and Endocrine Responses With Age

Two groups of hormones affect behavior. The first group—the catecholamines—act in two different ways. When released centrally, they function directly as neurotransmitters to affect neuronal control. Peripherally, they are released into the blood from the adrenal gland in response to stress. Epinephrine, norepinephrine, and dopamine are the three primary catecholamines involved in central and peripheral responses to stress.

The second group of hormones are related to the hypothalamic-anterior pituitary-adrenal axis. The adrenocortical axis refers to the hormonal connection between the corticotropin-releasing factor (CRF), which is produced in the hypothalamus; the adrenocorticotropic hormone (ACTH), which is produced

Table 10–1. Motor performance and cerebellar beta-adrenergic function of mature (10-month) and old (27-month) C57Bl mice

	10-month mice	27-month mice
Photobeam breaks	902 ± 47	583 ± 50*
Plank balance score	4.0 ± 0.4	2.3 ± 0.2*
Open field activity (rearing and loco-motion/10 min)	37.8 ± 1.3	21.2 ± 1.7*
Sitting (inactivity/10 min)	2.6 ± 0.5	16.2 ± 2.0*
Grooming (5 min)	1.3 ± 0.4	2.3 ± 0.6
Beta-receptor density (fmol/mg protein)	9.2 ± 0.1	20.0 ± 2.0*

*$P < .01$.

in the pituitary gland and is stimulated by CRF; and the glu-cocorticoids, which are produced in the adrenal gland, are stimulated by ACTH, and inhibit CRF.

Central Catecholamine Control of Motor Activity

Dopamine.   Of age changes in motor function, most promi-nent are decreases in motility and velocity (Janicke et al. 1983). Decreases in stimulated activity are not surprising because many movements are controlled by the basal ganglia, and it is well-known that aging alters central monoaminergic function (Roth 1983). Such neurotransmitter changes are most prominent in the basal ganglia and mesolimbic systems. Dopamine metabolism in the nucleus accumbens, a region receiving dense projections from the basal ganglia, is strongly linked to the speed of movement (Freed and Yamamoto 1985). Losing such terminals that project onto the mesolimbic system has been shown to impair motor response rates (Liljequist 1978). Consistent with the above findings, Marshall and Ber-rios (1979) showed that some of the motor defects of older rodents can be reversed by administration of dopaminergic agonists. Therefore, changes in motor function with age are related to decreases in the neuronal synthesis of dopamine (Watanabe 1987).

In addition to blunted neurotransmitter dynamics, there are also age-related differences in the physiological response to dopamine. Stimulation of locomotion by local injection of dopamine into the nucleus accumbens decreases with age (Cousin et al. 1986). This is consistent with diminished recep-tor function, as has been reported most notably in the striatum (Joseph et al. 1983a, 1983b). Dopamine receptor number decreases without a loss of affinity. Hence, defects at multiple levels in the neurotransmitter pathways are implicated in impaired motor responses with age. In summary, dopaminergic systems are markedly impaired with age; total levels as well as response patterns diminish, and this contributes to age-related alterations in motor function.

Norepinephrine. Norepinephrine networks change with age, but the changes are less dramatic than those in the dopaminergic system. Central nervous system levels of norepinephrine decline in a site-specific manner with aging (Finch 1973). The turnover of catecholamines in response to stressful stimuli also declines with age (Welsh and Gold 1984). However, the physiological significance of such changes is confounded by age-related shifts in synthesis (Ponzio et al. 1978) and metabolism (Robinson 1975).

Given this confusing picture in assessing age-related differences in presynaptic catecholamine production and metabolism, we elected to measure postsynaptic function (Rosenthal et al. 1988). Norepinephrine acts primarily by binding to a particular receptor subtype that subsequently activates neurochemical processes within selected cells. Age-related declines in beta-receptor number have been reported in cortex (Kohno et al. 1986), striatum (Maggi et al. 1979), and cerebellum (Pittman et al. 1980). We found that beta-receptor density but not receptor affinity was higher in cerebellum of 10-month than in 27-month C57Bl mice. These differences were well correlated to motor changes. In particular, receptor number was correlated to novelty-induced locomotion in an open field as well as to relatively nonstressed activity measured in a photocell box (Rosenthal et al. 1988). These results are consistent with the findings that postsynaptic responses to norepinephrine, including electrophysiological stimulation (Marawaha et al. 1980) and activation of adenylate cyclase (Walker and Walker 1973), are impaired with age.

Peripheral Catecholamines in Old Age

Catecholamines are potent hormones that can induce hypertension and spasm of essential blood supply when released peripherally. Chiueh et al. (1980), but not McCarty (1981, 1984), reported age-associated increases of basal plasma epinephrine or norepinephrine between young and old Fischer rats.

Adrenocortical Axis in Old Age

Corticosterone is the predominant glucocorticoid in rodents. Corticosterone-binding sites in the hippocampus are lost with age in rats (Sapolsky et al. 1983b) but not consistently in mice (Nelson et al. 1976). Studies comparing basal levels in older animals to levels in younger animals have produced contradictory results (Algeri et al. 1982; Grad and Khalid 1968; Sapolsky et al. 1983a; Scaccianoce et al. 1990). Differences in findings may reflect changes in response to diurnal rhythm. For example, DeKosky et al. (1984), but not Sonntag et al. (1988), found higher corticosterone levels at 6 P.M. and 11 P.M. in older compared with younger animals.

Yet, Sonntag et al. (1987) did find an age-related difference in the secretion of ACTH; the peak level declined during the diurnal surge (at 5 P.M.) when compared with younger rats (Sonntag et al. 1987). ACTH and beta-endorphin, which are coproduced and coreleased, both decline with aging in discrete brain areas, notably the hypothalamus and striatum (Gambert et al. 1980). Yet, the elevated basal plasma concentrations of beta-endorphin in old rats that have been reported may result from higher levels in the anterior and neurointermediate lobes of the pituitary (Forman et al. 1985; Missale et al. 1983).

Neuroendocrine stimulation is impaired at a number of levels with advanced age. Intravenous injection of CRF leads to smaller increases in corticosterone and ACTH for 20-month rats compared with young animals (Hylka et al. 1984). Central injection of CRF (5 μg) acts on different, predominantly autonomic, pathways, and such stimulation increases both plasma glucose and corticosterone to the same extent in 10- and 27-month mice (Rosenthal and Morley 1989). This response occurred despite the fact that elevations were sustained far longer than with somatic and psychological stressors (Figure 10–1).

Stimulation of hypothalamic CRF content is also diminished with age (Verkhratski et al. 1990), but some have reported increased release of bioactive CRF from hypothalamic blocks in culture (Scaccianoce et al. 1990). More distally the responses are also blunted.

Stress-Related Behaviors and Hormonal Responses

Experimental Rodent Behaviors During Stress

Both rats and mice display certain predictable behaviors when exposed to environmental challenges. These can be divided into groups of behaviors: exploration, avoidance, and anxiety.

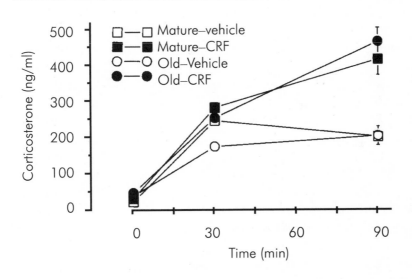

Figure 10–1.   Control of steroid release with age.
Source.   Reprinted from Rosenthal MJ, Morley JE: "Corticotropin Releasing Factor (CRF) and Age-Related Differences in Behavior of Mice." *Neurobiology of Aging* 10:167–171, 1989. Copyright 1989 by Pergamon Press.

Other behaviors, most notably feeding, cease with stress. When stressed, animals may not eat at all despite experiencing severe hunger.

During stress, rodents tend to walk or to rear on their hind legs. They often seek physical contact with others of the same species and tend to prefer dark quiet areas. If alone, rodents tend to groom and clean themselves. Under extreme stress, squealing, defecation, and urination as well as self-mutilation occur.

Hormonal Reactions to Stress

Adrenal activation prepares the body to fight or flee. Catecholamines and glucocorticoids mobilize energy resources by liberating fuels from storage depots. Glucocorticoids increase glucose production by stimulating gluconeogenesis and glycogenolysis. They bolster cardiovascular tone, maintain muscular work capacity, stimulate appetite, and promote hematopoiesis (Darlington et al. 1990). Cognition is acutely improved, and pain perception is blunted. Glucocorticoids also turn off nonessential processes as a means of optimizing survival during an emergency. Recently, it has come to be recognized that the immunosuppressant activity of these hormones may serve to prevent the development of autoimmunity when self-antigens are exposed by trauma. Thus, glucocorticoids play an important role in maintaining physiology under stress.

Neuropeptide Control: CRF Promotes Stress Behavior

Several other neurotransmitters are also involved in behavioral selection. CRF has a high degree of potency in releasing ACTH (corticotropin) from the anterior pituitary, hence the origin of its name. Yet, CRF is also widely distributed throughout the central nervous system (Rivier et al. 1982). Indeed, CRF appears to be an important regulator of several components of the stress response. It is found in sites outside the brain and has direct effects on the adrenal gland. Centrally administered CRF elicits a stress-like activation of the central monoaminergic system, and stress-induced elevation of catecholamines is blocked by a specific CRF antagonist (Dunn and Berridge 1987). Intraventricular, but not peripheral, administration of CRF enhances behavioral responses to novelty and elicits the expression of stress-like behavior of rats tested in their home cages (D. R. Britton et al. 1982). Specifically, such animals show increased grooming and decreased food consumption. Locomotor activity is also increased when rats are in their home environment, although such activity is decreased by CRF in a novel setting. Novelty-induced grooming may be a consequence of release of either ACTH (Gispen et al. 1975) or CRF (D. R. Britton et al. 1982). However, part of the response to CRF is not dependent on stimulation of ACTH. Neither hypophysectomy (Morley and Levine 1981) nor dexamethasone pretreatment (D. R. Britton et al. 1986) alters the behavioral actions of CRF. This suggests that those behavioral effects are mediated through direct neural pathways as opposed to hormonal. The parallel between responses elicited by CRF and those provoked by stressful stimuli suggests that endogenous CRF is one factor in stress-induced behaviors.

In summary, the administration of CRF replicates much but not all of behavioral and hormonal response to stress.

Interaction of Stress and Age-Related Changes

Age-Related Behavioral Responses to Stress

Environmental novelty: exploratory behaviors.   Placement in a new location represents mild stress. Both locomotion and rearing are less frequent in old compared with young animals during exposure to a novel environment (Sprott and Eleftheriou 1974). These age-dependent differences are affected by a number of factors, including group versus single testing, stimulus intensity (Goodrick 1975), temperature, and repeated exposure (Goodrick 1971). Brennan et al. (1982) reported lower exploratory behavior in 28-month versus 4- to 8-month mice; however, that behavior increased in the old rats with repeated prior exposure to the test apparatus and with prior restraint in a metal mesh envelope (Ritter 1978).

In summary, older rodents explore a novel setting less than young animals.

Grooming behaviors. Behaviors in response to stress other than rearing and locomotion are also changed with age. Grooming has been described as a displacement activity for lowering a state of high arousal (Kametani et al. 1984); it occurs in states of low arousal and increases during mild stress. Opiates and dopaminergic systems control grooming; haloperidol reduces grooming, and naloxone decreases both novelty- and ACTH-induced grooming. Some (Kametani et al. 1984), but not all (Jolles et al. 1979), investigators have found that the amount of novelty-induced grooming is greater in older compared with younger rats. During 50 minutes in an open field, 26-month Fischer rats showed more grooming bouts than 8-month rats, and each individual grooming bout was prolonged (Kametani et al. 1984). Jolles et al. observed no age difference in habituation to repeated exposure to stress.

Selection of behavior. We examined the pattern of selection of behaviors during stress by exposing rodents to a novel environment (Rosenthal et al. 1989). Rats of various ages were put in a situation of potential conflict by being partially food deprived before being placed in a well-lit open field in the center of which a single preweighed food pellet was secured. All rats, ages 3, 12, and 24 months, showed behavioral and hormonal stress responses when exposed to the novelty of the open field. Yet, there were marked age-dependent differences in behavior, which did not occur on the first day of testing, but only after repeated exposure (Figure 10–2). When rats were placed every day for 10 minutes into the open field, habituation of exploratory behavior as indicated by declining stress-responsive behaviors occurred far more rapidly in 24-month-old rats than in 3-month-old animals. The selection of behavior differed with age. Rearing, which is an exploratory behavior, increased less in old than in young rats. Conversely, grooming, which is a displacement behavior, increased with age (Figure 10–2).

In summary, old rodents select a different set of behaviors in response to stress than do young animals: grooming over exploration. These differences might be modulated by changes in central catecholamine pathways.

Age-Related Hormonal Responses to Stress

Central catecholamines.   Response of central catecholamines to stressors changes with age. Synthesis of hippocampal norepinephrine increases during restraint stress to a greater extent in old than in young rats (Algeri et al. 1988), and recovery of stress-induced increases in norepinephrine turnover is delayed (Ida et al. 1984). Conversely, stress increases striatal dopamine and its precursors less (Algeri et al. 1988), but serotonin precursors more (Algeri et al. 1982), in old than in young rats. As discussed earlier, aging is associated with decreases in beta-receptor number. Moreover, the adaptive response of this system to stress is blunted. Receptor number down-regulates in young but not old rats after 60 minutes of immobilization stress, and redistribution of surface receptors is similarly lost with aging (De Blasi et al. 1987). Finally, hypothalamic norepinephrine concentrations were higher in rats able to escape foot-shock stress than in rats unable to escape, whereas hippocampal norepinephrine decreased only in coping rats once they learned to terminate foot shock (Swenson and Vogel 1983). In this way, rats who are unable to escape resemble older rats.

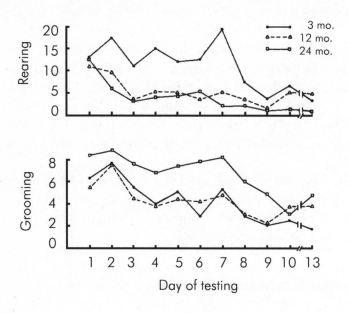

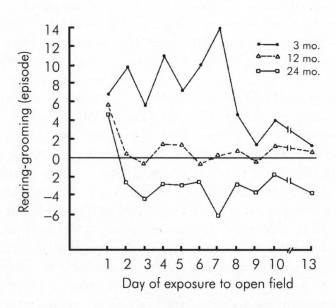

Figure 10–2.   Open field behavior of aging rodents.

Peripheral catecholamines.   Chiueh et al. (1980) noted greater catecholamine increases after 30 minutes of immobilization stress in old than young rats, whereas McCarty (1981) found that foot-shock–induced increments of norepinephrine and epinephrine were 38% and 63% lower, respectively, in older animals. Differences in findings between these two studies may be due to the shorter recovery time after cannulae placement by Chiueh et al. The increase in epinephrine, norepinephrine, and mean arterial blood pressure did not differ between 12- and 24-month Fischer 344 rats during nonexertional heat stress. However, norepinephrine response was higher in 6- versus 24-month rats, and epinephrine was higher in the older rats after 2-deoxyglucose (McCarty 1984). During recovery, the declines toward control were similar or more rapid in the older rats (Kegel et al. 1990). Others reported a greater increase in the catecholamine response to stress in 16- than in 4-month-old rats (Taylor et al. 1989).

In summary, there is contradictory evidence concerning whether there is a greater peripheral catecholamine response to stress in older compared with younger rodents.

The toxic effects of vasoconstriction due to catecholamines does increase with age. There is an age-related increase in release of tissue enzymes after restraint in rats (Rattner et al. 1983). Exposure to electric foot shock for 6 minutes on 3 successive days increased adrenal tyrosine hydroxylase activity, the rate-limiting enzyme for catecholamine production, in 1- but not in 12-month rats. This deficit in older rats was overcome by prior exposure to the stress of electric foot shock, presumably via reduction of the magnitude of the corticosterone response, which leads to an increase in tyrosine hydroxylase activity (Pfeifer and Davis 1975).

Prolonged catecholamine and corticosterone elevations as have been reported for older rats also occur in rats exposed to inescapable foot shock. The inability to cope augments both plasma catecholamine and corticosterone increases in responses to a stressor and prolongs their return to baseline (Swenson and Vogel 1983). These responses can be modulated by early life events. For example, injection of L-dopa during early ontogeny, day 24, which elevates brain but not peripheral catecholamines, promotes a long-lasting decrease of stress-induced blood pressure (Naumenko et al. 1990).

Catecholamines elevate glucose and free fatty acids in part by suppressing insulin release. Hence age changes in catecholamine function have physiological repercussions. Epinephrine (Dax et al. 1981) and other hormone-stimulated lipolysis (Hoffman et al. 1984) decreases in older adipocytes, and this is changed by dietary intervention (Yu et al. 1980). Electric shock increased metabolic fuels more in 6- than in 24-month Fischer 344 rats (Odio and Brodish 1988).

In summary, changes in catecholamine production responses with age vary between experiments but regardless, the toxic, often fatal, response to catecholamines is excessive in older rodents.

Adrenal response.   There are a number of alterations in the adrenal response. Chronic (21-day) hypoxic stress, presumably through pituitary-enhanced adrenal capacity, augments the ACTH-stimulated steroid production of cultured adrenal cells from young but not from old rats (Cheng et al. 1990). ACTH stimulation of corticosterone response is impaired in vivo (Hess and Riegle 1970) and in vitro in old rodents (Malamed and Carsia 1983; E. Reaven et al. 1988). The site of the defect appears to be distal to the binding of the tropic hormone to its plasma membrane receptor and to the production of its second messenger (Popplewell et al. 1986).

Advanced age does not diminish the rapidity of the rise and the maximum corticosterone level after most stressors. Although we found exploratory activity to be less in old rodents during exposure to a novel open field, we found no age difference in plasma corticosterone increases after 30 minutes of such stressful exposure (Rosenthal et al. 1989) (see Table 10–2). This agreed with the results of Eleftheriou (1974), but was contrary to the lower maximal levels reported in older female rats (Brett et al. 1986).

Several others have reported a significantly smaller corticosterone response with advanced age to ether, a severe stressor (Brett et al. 1981; Hess and Riegle 1970; Wilson et al. 1981); this decrease occurs despite the fact that ether, being fat soluble, presumably persists longer in older rats than in younger rats because older rats are more obese. Starvation also led to lower corticosterone responses in old rats (G. W. Britton et al. 1975). Reserve capacity also appears to be unchanged in that older rats respond normally to novelty when exposed after previous chronic stress (Sapolsky et al. 1983a). This was the situation when we repeatedly exposed rats to the novelty of an open field; even after 14 days there was still no age difference in corticosterone response (Rosenthal et al. 1989). In contrast, Riegel (1973) found that corticosterone response to chronic restraint decreased with repeated stress for all rats. Despite twice daily restraint for 20 days, old female rats, but not old male or young rats, continued to show hormonal elevation. Prior restraint decreased corticosterone response to ether less in old than in young rats. (However, response to repeated stress may be impaired.) Odio and Brodish (1989b) found that corticosterone responses were higher in old rats on the third but not on the first day of shock.

The older pituitary-adrenal axis can respond effectively to a mild stress, although fast feedback inhibition is impaired

Table 10–2. Plasma immunoreactive corticosterone (μg/dl) under basal (home cage) and stimulated (2 weeks of daily exposure to open field) conditions in Fischer 344 rats

	Age (months)		
Condition	3	12	24
Home cage	8.7 ± 1.0	10.5 ± 1.6	7.9 ± 1.0
Open field	16.7 ± 1.3	15.3 ± 1.2	13.6 ± 1.4

Note. Open field levels were significantly higher than home cage values for each age group ($P < .05$; $n = 10$ per age group). There were no significant differences across age groups.

(Sapolsky et al. 1986a). Suppression by endogenous corticosterone was also reported to be impaired after chronic restraint
(Riegel 1973). Repeated stress decreased the corticosterone
response to chronic injection of ACTH to a greater degree in
young than in old rats (Hess et al. 1970). Tang and Phillips
(1978) extended these results by measuring ACTH levels
immediately after ether (2.5 or 15 minutes) and following recovery (12.5 minutes). Shorter stress led to equivalent
responses but prolonged stress produced a 100-fold increase in
plasma ACTH levels in young rodents (2.5 and 7.5 months)
versus a lesser, only 15-fold, increase in older animals (12, 18,
and 26 months). However, 90% recovery to basal levels
occurred in young rats over the 12.5-minute study, and no
recovery was observed in the older rats, which also showed
higher basal levels.

Age-related decrements were reported in suppression of
stress-induced adrenal activation after chronic or acute dexamethasone in male and in female rats (Oxenkrug et al. 1984;
Riegel and Hess 1972). In vitro, dexamethasone inhibition of
ACTH release from quartered anterior pituitaries did not show
age changes (Scaccianoce et al. 1990).

In summary, although corticosterone responses to stress are
well sustained in older rodents, central control of the adrenal-
pituitary axis is impaired in older animals. For instance, ACTH
responses to psychological and somatic stressors are decreased
in 6- versus 24-month F344 rats.

Yet, the capacity of CRF and ACTH to respond to stress in
old rodents can be improved by manipulating the environment. The greatest capacity of the adrenal to secrete corticosteroids occurs at levels of ACTH between 150 and 300 pg/ml,
and such levels can be achieved by old animals. Deficient
ACTH responses of old rats can be reversed by daily repeated
foot shock over 6 months (Odio and Brodish 1989). Such
chronic stress led to increased corticosterone response to novelty in young but not in old rats, presumably because of adrenal impairment. Environmental factors may delay the
development of age-related physiological alterations in the

pituitary-adrenocortical system. Exercise increases cold tolerance in old rats (McDonald et al. 1988).

Role of CRF in Age Changes of Behavior

Though age-related changes in cerebellar noradrenergic pathways and mesolimbic and nucleus accumbens dopaminergic
systems might well explain differences in locomotion during
open field exposure, the lack of consistent differences in basal
(i.e., home cage) behavior suggests that stress-related factors
are involved. Certainly, several different classes of neurotransmitters produce behavioral activation. Sympathomimetics,
methylxanthines, opiates, and several neuropeptides are
chemically distinct. Using photocell-measured motor activity
in rats, Swerdlow et al. (1986) found that certain of these
behavioral activating neurochemicals act on common neural
substrates. Other agents act on seemingly distinct brain regions. Sympathomimetics and opiates seem to act primarily
within the basal ganglia. Contrarily, caffeine and CRF act on a
separate circuit.

The lack of major age-related differences in behavioral
responses to CRF suggests that the locomotor activating properties of CRF are distinct from the effects of sympathomimetics and opiates, which act primarily in the basal ganglia.
Although responses to CRF did not appear to explain age differences in behavior, endogenous activation has not been studied. However, age-related differences in response to other
neurotransmitters have been reported. Open field activity of
older rats was unaffected by morphine in doses that activated
young rats; similar results were found after subcutaneous injection of methadone (Middaugh et al. 1983). Young mice (6–
8 months) demonstrated greater motor activation than 30- to
32-month mice. Inability of older rodents to move as rapidly
as younger animals is likely to have played a major role in these
differences as well as in the lack of correction of deficits by
CRF. Thus, *motor* changes that can be modified by neurotrans-

mitters such as dopamine seem to override age differences in *behavioral* responsivity to stressors.

The notion of a separate pathway for behavioral activation and the parallels between stress-responsive behaviors and the response to intracerebroventricular (ICV) injection of CRF prompted our studies of centrally administered CRF in older rodents. Mice age 10 months, mature, and 27 months were injected ICV with varying doses of CRF (Rosenthal and Morley 1989). Open field behavior differed significantly between groups. Older mice reared less and were more likely to sit and be immobile or to groom. Old mice stayed near the location where they were initially placed. CRF decreased feeding but this response was not affected by age. Neither was there any reversal of the age-related differences in locomotion after injection of CRF. Thus, CRF does not reverse age deficits in stress-induced behavior. A possible defect in CRF in older rats does not explain the decrease in behavioral response to stress in older animals.

Age Changes in Other Stress-Responsive Hormones

This discussion emphasizes glucocorticoids because these hormones seem to play the largest role in the process of aging. Nevertheless, there are age-related changes in the response of other pituitary hormones (Forman et al. 1981). Secretion of prolactin and growth hormone increase in response to numerous stressors (Brown and Martin 1974; Kant et al. 1983). Thyrotropin also is released in parallel with growth hormone (Armario and Garcia-Marquez 1987) and, as with ACTH, the acute rise is blunted after chronic stress (Keller-Wood et al. 1983). The thyroid-stimulating hormone response is complex and may not be as good an indicator of the stress as other hormones. For example, thyroid-stimulating hormone release was increased 10 minutes after immobilization but decreased by 30 minutes (Armario and Jolin 1989). The effects of aging on this pattern have not been studied.

Prolactin. Prolactin increases after different stressors than ACTH. Restraint and surgery but not cold stress increase prolactin (Donnerer and Lembeck 1990). We have found that plasma prolactin increases fivefold after foot shock and that responses follow a course parallel that for corticosterone (Ratner et al. 1989). Although mice show no age-related changes in basal circulating levels of immunoreactive prolactin (Finch et al. 1977), levels are reported to increase in aging male rats (Bethea and Walker 1979). However, basal bioactive prolactin levels were lower in old rats (Briski and Sylvester 1990). Inhibition of prolactin by methyldopa is blunted and delayed in both male and female old rats (Riegel and Meites 1976) as is the decrease after naltrexone (Briski and Sylvester 1991). However, there was no apparent age difference in the prolactin increase after the stress of unaccustomed handling and intraperitoneal injection. Thirty minutes of restraint stress increased prolactin to the same amount in 3-month (cycling) and 26-month rats (Demarest et al. 1987). Despite these findings, Briski and Sylvester (1990) reported that levels of *immunoreactive* prolactin increased normally in old rats exposed to strobe lights or restraint but that the response of *bioactive* hormone decreased significantly with age. In contrast to corticosterone, there were no age differences in response to ether.

In summary, prolactin responds to stress in different ways than glucocorticoids in young rats but shows relatively little age change in pattern of response to stress.

Luteinizing hormone. The luteinizing hormone response to stress is far less in older than in younger animals. Methyldopa stimulates luteinizing hormone elevations in young but not in old rats. Stressful exposure increases plasma luteinizing hormone levels dramatically, almost fivefold, in young rats after cage disturbance, but there is no increase in levels for 30-month Long Evans rats.

Growth hormone. Prolactin is often linked to growth hormone response by similarities of stimulation (Demarest et al.

1987). There are similar age changes with decreased gene expression (messenger RNA production) of both prolactin and growth hormone in older mouse pituitaries (Crew et al. 1987). However, growth hormone shows divergent patterns during stress (Brown and Martin 1974). Growth hormone dynamics that change considerably in older humans also change with aging in rodents (Sonntag et al. 1983). Contrary to the case for gonadotropins, methyldopa corrects some of the defects in amplitude of growth hormone pulses in old male rats (Sonntag et al. 1982). However, stress-related processes as replicated by adrenal stimulation and morphine injection lead to decreased growth hormone responses in older rodents (Sonntag et al. 1980). Despite decreased release after surgical stress (Cartlidge et al. 1970), growth hormone responses to the stress of hypoglycemia are preserved at advanced age (Blichert-Toft 1975).

The role of acute responses of these stress-responsive hormones is not always clear. Prolactin regulates lactation and has a luteotropic action on the rat ovary, but the role in males and as part of the stress response is unclear. The largest population of pituitary cells even in old animals are those that produce growth hormone. Although the physiological part played by growth hormone is unclear in older animals, it is metabolically active and may serve an anabolic function at advanced age.

How Age Leads to Less Active Stress Responses: Hypotheses

Aging alters certain behaviors in response to stress. A major portion of this change relates to age deficits in neurotransmitter function. Such changes in behavior are corroborated by age changes in the patterns of hormonal response to stress. Blunted physiological capacity may cause such changes.

Disruption of neural and endocrine function may contribute to the reduced ability of older animals to adapt and, in extreme situations, to survive exposure to stress (Pare 1965). Their impaired recovery from stress exposure may explain why older mice showed prolonged activation after cold-swim stress (Thurmond and Heishman 1984). Either deficient or excessive responses with aging may explain why the capacity to maintain internal homeostasis is impaired (Timiras 1978).

Impaired Steroid Feedback Dynamics

In order to maintain metabolic homeostasis, the hypotha-lamic-anterior pituitary-adrenal axis must perform within constraints regulated by negative feedback systems. Not only must the axis be able to stimulate release of glucocorticoids in response to stressful events, but it must also be able to shut itself off when the need no longer exists. Rising glucocorticoid levels act to inhibit ACTH release from the anterior pituitary. Steroids also act on the hypothalamus and higher structures, most notably the hippocampus. Glucocorticoids alter receptor function at both levels, which, in turn, modulates feed for-ward pathways. Advanced age may lead to defects in these feedback controls.

A portion of the age-related disparity may derive from senescent effects on lability of the adrenal-pituitary axis (Brett et al. 1986). Corticosterone is entrained by restriction of food or of water, but old female rats failed to reentrain or to sup-press corticosterone secretion on drinking and did not exhibit increased levels with food deprivation (Brett et al. 1986). Al-though young rats began to show a decrease in corticosterone after reaching a peak at 2 hours, older rats continued to in-crease levels even after 24-hour exposure to cold (Algeri et al. 1982). Impaired capacity to sustain homeostasis may have led to prolonged elevation of stress hormones. Such was the case with prolonged cold exposure; senescent rats were unable to compensate for loss of body heat (Algeri et al. 1982). Some investigators have noted that older rats recover more slowly after stressful stimulation, and this may lead to persistently elevated steroid levels of moderate degree, which in turn may lead to blunted ACTH and CRF stimulation of corticosterone.

In recent years, support for the role of excess steroids in this cascade of aging pathology has been most prominently advocated by Sapolsky and by Landfield. Sapolsky found that peak corticosterone responses to stressors were unchanged but that elevated levels persist for at least 60 minutes longer in old than in young rats after immobilization (Sapolsky et al. 1983a). Others found elevated corticosterone after various stressors. Such findings could have many explanations, including 1) decreased metabolic clearance of glucocorticoids as occurs in humans, which is not observed in rodents (E. Reaven et al. 1988); 2) impaired physiological recovery from stress, which definitely occurs; or 3) lost glucocorticoid feedback inhibition, which probably happens.

Aging dramatically alters the stress-responsive cascade by down-regulating glucocorticoid receptors and ultimately decreasing neuronal control at the hippocampus (Sapolsky et al. 1983b). This brain region is essential to both feed forward and feed backward systems of adrenal steroids. Histopathological hippocampal aging is also correlated to age and elevation of cumulative exposure to glucocorticoids (Landfield et al. 1978). Diurnal corticosterone levels in older rats are sufficient to reduce neural recovery as measured by lesion-induced axonal sprouting (DeKosky et al. 1984). In other words, after experimental destruction of nerves, regrowth of those nerves that often starts from the axons (i.e., the essential conducting fibers of the nerve fiber) is impaired by corticosterone.

Regulation of hippocampal steroid receptors is also blunted with age. The hippocampus and the septal areas are primary target sites for corticosterone (Knizley 1972). Stress-induced decreases in receptors are impaired (Eldridge et al. 1989a) and so are adrenalectomy-induced increases (Eldridge et al. 1989b).

The hippocampal changes are also involved in cognitive aging (Landfield 1988). Issa et al. (1990) found that healthy old rats with mildly impaired spatial memory had greater neuron loss in the pyramidal cell fields of the hippocampus. This group of animals also demonstrated higher basal levels of corticosterone and ACTH as well as impaired hormonal recovery after restraint.

Stressful events during infancy, such as withdrawal from the mother and isolation, lead to the same loss of hippocampal steroid receptors that develops with advanced age. This abnormality persists throughout life and leads to elevated glucocorticoid responses to stressors (Dennenberg and Zarrow 1971; Levine and Mullins 1966). Hence, there may be behaviors that promote loss of essential steroid receptors and ultimate cognitive impairment; these decrements may be linked by the loss of adequate steroid termination mechanisms.

The relevance of these exaggerated steroid responses begins to become clear. It has been hypothesized that aging may, in part, be caused by impaired hysteresis; that is, heightened responses of neuropeptides may over time blunt the response to subsequent stimulation. In essence, this means that the ultimate response is diminished even though the initial defect was an excessive response.

Although the stimulation of the steroid axis seems to be relatively unchanged with advanced age, in certain situations, the steroid responses are actually too robust in older rodents. This excessive response may relate to the fact that the feedback system is damaged with advanced age. Sapolsky (1984a) found that this may in part explain the steroid abnormalities.

In summary, the steroid axis is controlled through receptors that diminish with age. This diminution may explain the occurrence of impaired feedback recovery in old rodents.

Comparison of Aging and Chronic Stress

Aging might be viewed as a chronic inescapable stress comparable with that from which a posttraumatic stress disorder originates. Giving daily repeated foot shock with a randomly altered duration and interval between shocks to modestly restrained rats was used as a model of such stress. This chronic shock resulted in decreased exploratory activity, especially decreased rearing, as is found in older rats. Immobility was also prolonged during forced swim (Garcia-Marquez and Armario 1987). However, hormonal responses after chronic stress did not follow aging patterns. The ACTH response was unchanged to subsequent absolute immobilization or to environmental novelty. Results were similar when chronic variable stress was tested in which different stressors were administered each day at different times for 24 days (Garcia-Marquez and Armario 1987). This does not explain the lowered ACTH observed in older animals, which presumably relates to inhibition from intermittently elevated glucocorticoids (Keller-Wood and Bell 1988). It is possible that there is a critical interval during which stressful events catalyze aging events. Sapolsky et al. (1986b) found that exposure to stress in early life so alters the neurophysiology of an animal that aging changes irrevocably occur at an excessive rate.

In summary, impaired steroid recovery with advanced age may relate to previous stressful responses.

Stress Responses and Acute Illness

Although nonmaximal physiological hormone responses are preserved with advanced age, this is not the situation with acute illness, which has many other features similar to aging. When rats developed pneumonia, basal levels of corticosterone were elevated twofold but the response to subsequent electric shock was absolutely suppressed in sick rats. Healthy rats increased plasma corticosterone from 10 to 55 μg/dl and prolactin from 10 to 45 ng/ml, but there was absolutely no change in either prolactin or corticosterone level in acutely ill rats (Yelvington et al. 1987). Not all types of acute illness lead to this blunting of the stress response. Indeed acute diabetes induced by streptozotocin with dehydration and sky-high glucose levels causes a state of elevated corticosterone in which the subsequent response to stressors is exaggerated (Rhees et al. 1983); this is corrected by insulin treatment. Diabetes out of control promotes dehydration that induces release of another stress hormone, vasopressin, which in turn acts to stimulate corticotropin release. The mechanism for the persistent heightened glucocorticoid response of diabetic rodents involves loss of hippocampal glucocorticoid receptors (Tornello et al. 1981) as occurs with age, and it may relate to vasopressin induction of CRF message. Aging also induces a state of excess vasopressin release (Miller 1987), which may be involved in altered adrenal-pituitary feedback control.

Detrimental Responses to Life-Saving Hormones

Selye first described the two-edged sword of hormonal responses to stress. Although adrenal hormones are critical to survival, when released in overabundance or for prolonged periods they can be deleterious. These essential hormones lead to a cascade of toxic reactions. Many of the toxic responses to stressors seem to lie in the glucocorticoid response (Munck et al. 1984; Okwusidi et al. 1991).

Parallels have been drawn between the pathology of Cushing's disease and of aging (Wexler 1978). Excessive glucocorticoids create a Cushingoid state characterized by glucose intolerance, hyperlipidemia, high blood pressure, central obesity, immune dysfunction (Fauci and Dale 1974), atherosclerosis, and cognitive impairment (Bulkey and Roberts 1975; Kalbak 1972). As in the aging process, catabolic processes are accelerated in skeletal muscle and skin (David et al. 1970). Furthermore, chronic glucocorticoid excess increases the incidence of vascular disease in humans and induces atherosclerotic lesion in animals in the absence of hyperlipidemia (Wexler 1978). The range of pathological conditions induced by corticosteroid excess is not unlike that seen during the course of human aging (Table 10–3). This pattern occurs floridly in the death of anadromous fish, notably salmon. During migration upstream, acute steroid excess develops, causing rapid senescence and death due to catabolism marked by atherosclerosis and fungal infections (Everitt 1976). Although this example of fulminant glucocorticoid intoxication is exaggerated, there are remarkable parallels between states of glucocorticoid excess and aging.

The deleterious role of endogenous glucocorticoid responses is also supported by the beneficial effects of hypophysectomy. Removing the anterior pituitary in the young rat retards a number of physiological age changes: collagen aging in rat tail tendon, the incidence of tumors, and age-related progression of renal failure and proteinuria. Many of these improvements are similar to the benefit from dietary restriction (Ingram et al. 1987). Nevertheless, life span is increased by dietary restriction and contrarily is shortened by hypophysec-

Table 10–3.   Analogy between Cushingoid state and aging

Cushing's	Aging
Myopathy	Loss of lean body mass
Central obesity	Higher percentage of weight is fat; gynoid (central) pattern common
Glucose intolerance (occasional diabetes)	Glucose intolerance, 25% diabetes by age 70
Hypertension	Increased blood pressure almost universal with advanced age
Hyperlipidemia	Increased cholesterol and triglycerides with age
Depression	Depression more frequent with aging
Atherosclerosis	Nearly universal with age
Osteoporosis	Loss of bone matrix and calcium load with age
Immune dysfunction	T cell function impaired with age
Cognitive impairment	Benign senile forgetfulness
Protein wasting	Easy bruising, thinning skin with striae

Source.   Adapted from Liddle 1981.

tomy despite periodic treatments with physiological doses of cortisone (Everitt 1976).

In summary, glucocorticoids have a number of detrimental effects that in some species lead directly to death.

Conclusion

By and large, older animals are able to mount successful responses during stressful arousal despite the loss of certain components of that response. However, when faced with maximal stimulation, older animals manage poorly. Maximal responses are diminished, and mortality is increased. This response pattern occurs with a number of behavioral and hormonal indicators.

Aging may entail a combination of the discrepant hormonal mechanisms outlined for acute illness. Rather than a diminished corticosterone response to stressful stimuli in older rodents, the response is at least as great as in younger animals and may well be excessive.

Yet, aging is characterized by a blunted ability to correct homeostatic perturbations, which may be the explanation for some of the impairments of central stimulation. Aging impairs the physiological response to homeostatic challenges such as exercise, hypoxia, and high or low temperature (Rattner et al. 1983). Eating, drinking, and locomotion induced by hypoxia are decreased (Schulze and Janicke 1986). Cold temperature induces greater hypothermia, more weight loss, and higher mortality in older rats (McDonald et al. 1988).

The cumulative effects of stressful occurrences at younger ages may promote the development of much aging physiology and ultimately make the organism susceptible to death from an assault that could easily have been withstood. The hormonal and behavioral components of this deterioration are linked.

Chronic stress, or stress at critical windows of development, seems to promote many of the neurological deficits that comprise aging. There are certainly central nervous system re-percussions from such chronic stress. These impair the capacity to sustain homeostasis, and this deficit is central to what constitutes aging.

References

Algeri S, Calderini G, Lomuscio G, et al: Changes with age in rat central monoaminergic system responses to cold stress. Neurobiol Aging 3:237–242, 1982

Algeri S, Calderini G, Lomuscio B, et al: Differential response to immobilization stress of striatal dopaminergic and hippocampal noradrenergic systems in aged rats. Neurobiol Aging 9:213–216, 1988

Armario A, Garcia-Marquez C: The effects of chronic intermittent stress on basal and acute stress levels of TSH and GH, and their response to hypothalamic regulatory factors in the rat. Psychoneuroendocrinology 12:399–406, 1987

Armario A, Jolin TG: Influence of intensity and duration of exposure to various stressors on serum TSH and GH levels in adult male rats. Life Sci 44:215–221, 1989

Bethea CL, Walker RF: Age-related changes in reproductive hormones and in Leydig cell responsivity in the male Fisher 344 rat. J Gerontol 34:21–27, 1979

Blichert-Toft M: Secretion of corticotrophin and somatotrophin by the senescent adenohypophysis of man. Acta Endocrinol (Copenh) 78 (suppl 195):1–157, 1975

Brennan MJ, Blizard DA, Quartermain D: Amelioration of an age-related deficit in exploratory behavior by pre-exposure to the test environment. Behav Neural Biol 34:55–62, 1982

Brett LP, Levine R, Levine S: Bidirectional responsiveness of the pituitary-adrenal system in old and young male and female rats. Neurobiol Aging 7:153–159, 1983

Briski KP, Sylvester PW: Comparative effects of various stressors on immunoreactive versus bioactive prolactin release in old and young male rats. Neuroendocrinology 51:625–631, 1990

Briski KP, Sylvester PW: Effect of Naltrexone on stress-induced bioactive prolactin release in aging male rats. Neurobiol Aging 12:145–149, 1991

Britton DR, Koob GF, Rivier J, et al: Intraventricular corticotropin-releasing factor enhances behavioral effects of novelty. Life Sci 31:363–368, 1982

Britton DR, Varela M, Garcia A, et al: Dexamethasone suppresses the pituitary-adrenal but not the behavioral effects of centrally administered CRF. Life Sci 38:211–216, 1986

Britton GW, Rotenberg WS, Adelman RC: Impaired regulation of corticosterone levels during fasting in aging rats. Biochem Biophys Res Commun 64:184–188, 1975

Brown GM, Martin JB: Corticosterone, prolactin and growth hormone responses to handling and new environment in the rat. Psychosom Med 36:241–247, 1974

Bulkey BH, Roberts WC: The heart in systemic lupus and the changes induced by corticosteroid therapy. Am J Med 58:243–264, 1975

Cartlidge NEF, Black MM, Hall MRP, et al: Pituitary function in the elderly. Gerontologia Clinica 12:65–70, 1970

Cheng G, Horst IA, Mader SL, et al: Diminished adrenal steroidogenic activity in aging rats: new evidence from adrenal cells cultured from young and aged normal and hypoxic animals. Mol Cell Endocrinol 73:R7–R12, 1990

Chiueh CC, Nespor SM, Rapoport SI: Cardiovascular, sympathetic and adrenal cortical responsiveness of aged Fischer-344 rats to stress. Neurobiol Aging 1:157–163, 1980

Cousin KM, Gerald MC, Uretsky NJ: Effects of mialamide on the metabolism of dopamine injected into the nucleus accumbens of old rats. J Pharmacol Exp Ther 237:25–30, 1986

Crew MD, Spindler SR, Walford RC, et al: Age-related decrease of growth hormone and prolactin gene expression in the mouse pituitary. Endocrinology 121:1251–1255, 1987

Darlington DN, Chew G, Ha T, et al: Corticosterone, but not glucose, treatment enables fasted adrenalectomized rats to survive moderate hemorrhage. Endocrinology 127:766–772, 1990

David DS, Grieco H, Cushman P: Adrenal glucocorticoids after 20 years: a review of their clinically relevant consequences. J Chronic Dis 22:637–711, 1970

Dax EM, Partilla JS, Gregerman RI: Mechanism of the age-related decrease of epinephrine stimulated lipolysis in isolated rat adipocytes: β-adrenergic receptor binding, adenylate cyclase activity and cyclic AMP accumulation. J Lipid Res 22:934–943, 1981

De Blasi A, Fratelli M, Wielosz M, et al: Regulation of beta adrenergic receptors on rat mononuclear leukocytes by stress: receptor redistribution and down-regulation are altered with aging. J Pharmacol Exp Ther 240:228–233, 1987

DeKosky ST, Scheff SW, Cotman CW: Elevated corticosterone levels: a possible cause of reduced axons-sprouting in aged animals. Neuroendocrinology 38:33–38, 1984

Demarest KT, Moore KE, Riegel GD: Restraint stress decreases the neurosecretory activity of tuberoinfundibular dopaminergic neurons in young but not in aged female rats. Neuroendocrinology 45:333–337, 1987

Dennenberg VH, Zarrow MX: Effects of handling in infancy upon adult behavior and adrenocortical activity, in Early Childhood: The Development of Regulating Mechanisms. Edited by Walcher DN, Peters D. New York, Academic, 1971, pp 40–71

Donnerer J, Lembeck F: Different control of the adrenocorticotropin-corticosterone response and of prolactin secretion during cold stress, anesthesia, surgery and nicotine injection in the rat. Endocrinology 126:921–926, 1990

Dunn AJ, Berridge CW: CRF elicits a stress-like activation of cerebral catecholaminergic systems. Pharmacol Biochem Behav 27:1–6, 1987

Eldridge JC, Brodish A, Kute TE, et al: Apparent age-related resistance of type II hippocampal corticosteroid receptors to down-regulation during chronic escape training. J Neurosci 9:3237–3242, 1989a

Eldridge JC, Fleenor DG, Kerr DS, et al: Impaired up-regulation of type II corticosteroid receptors in hippocampus of aged rats. Brain Res 478:246–248, 1989b

Eleftheriou BE: Changes with age in adrenal-pituitary responsiveness and reactivity to mild stress in mice. Gerontologia 20:224–230, 1974

Everitt AV: Hypophysectomy and aging in the rat, in Hypothalamus Pituitary and Aging. Edited by Everitt AV, Burgess JA. Springfield, IL, Charles C Thomas, 1976, pp 66–86

Fauci AS, Dale DC: The effect of in vivo hydrocortisone on subpopulations of human lymphocytes. J Clin Invest 53:240–241, 1974

Finch CE: Catecholamine metabolism in the brains of aging male mice. Brain Res 52:261–276, 1973

Finch CE, Jones C, Wisner JR, et al: Hormone production by the pituitary and testes of male C57Bl/6J mice during aging. Endocrinology 101:1310–1317, 1977

Forman L, Sonntag W, Meites J: Immunoreactive beta-endorphin in the plasma, pituitary and hypothalamus of young and old male rats. Neurobiol Aging 2:281–285, 1981

Forman LJ, Marquis D, Stevens R: Release of immunoreactive beta-endorphin in vitro from pituitaries of young and old male rats. Neurobiol Aging 6:101–105, 1985

Freed CR, Yamamoto BK: Regional brain dopamine metabolism: a marker for speed, direction and posture of moving animals. Science 228:62–67, 1985

Gambert SR, Garthwaite TL, Pontzer CH, et al: Age-related changes in central nervous system beta-endorphin and ACTH. Neuroendocrinology 31:252–255, 1980

Garcia-Marquez A, Armario A: Chronic stress depresses exploratory activity and behavioral performance in the forced swimming test without altering ACTH response to a novel acute stressor. Physiol Behav 40:33–381, 1987

Gispen WH, Wiegant V, Greven H, et al: The induction of excessive grooming in the rat by intracerebroventricular application of peptides derived from ACTH. Life Sci 17:645–652, 1975

Goodrick CL: Free exploration and adaptation within an open field as a function of trials and between trial interval for mature-young, mature-old, and senescent Wistar rats. J Gerontol 26:58–62, 1971

Goodrick CL: Adaptation to novel environments by the rat: effects of age, stimulus intensity, group testing and temperature. Developmental Psychology 8:287–296, 1975

Grad B, Khalid R: Circulating coticosterone levels of young and old male and female C5761 mice. J Gerontol 23:522–528, 1968

Hess GD, Riegle GD: Adrenocortical responsiveness to stress and ACTH in aging rats. J Gerontol 25:354–358, 1970

Hylka VW, Sonntag WE, Meites J: Reduced ability of old male rats to release ACTH and corticosterone in responses to CRF administration. Proc Soc Exp Biol Med 175:1–4, 1984

Ida Y, Tanaka M, Tsuda A, et al: Recovery of stress-induced increases in noradrenaline turnover is delayed in specific brain regions of old rats. Life Sci 34:2357–2360, 1984

Ingram DK, Weindruch R, Spangler EL, et al: Dietary restriction benefits learning and motor performance of aged mice. J Gerontol 42:76–81, 1987

Issa AM, Rowe W, Gauthier S, et al: Hypothalamic-pituitary-adrenal activity in aged, cognitively impaired and cognitively unimpaired rats. J Neurosci 10:3247–3254, 1990

Janicke B, Schultze G, Coper H: Motor performance achievement in rats of different ages. Exp Gerontol 18:393–407, 1983

Jolles J, Rompa-Barendregt J, Gispen WH: Novelty and grooming behavior in the rat. Behav Neural Biol 25:563–572, 1979

Joseph JA, Whitaker J, Roth GS, et al: Life-long dietary restriction affects striatally mediated behavioral responses in aged rats. Neurobiol Aging 4:191–196, 1983a

Joseph JA, Bartus RT, Clody D, et al: Psychomotor performance in the senescent rodent: reduction of deficits via striatal dopamine receptor up-regulation. Neurobiol Aging 4:313–319, 1983b

Kalbak K: Incidence of arteriosclerosis in patients with rheumatoid arthritis receiving long-term corticosteroid therapy. Ann Rheum Dis 31:196–200, 1972

Kametani H, Osada H, Inoue K: Increased novelty-induced grooming in aged rats. Behav Neural Biol 42:73–80, 1984

Kant GJ, Lenox RH, Runnell BN, et al: Comparison of stress response in male and female rats: pituitary cAMP and plasma prolactin, growth hormone and corticosterone. Psychoneuroendocrinology 8:421–428, 1983

Kegel KC, Johnson DG, Tipton CM, et al: Cardiovascular-sympathetic adjustments to nonexertional heat stress in mature and senescent Fischer 344 rats. J Appl Physiol 69:2043–2049, 1990

Keller-Wood M, Bell ME: Evidence for rapid inhibition of ACTH by corticosteroids in dogs. Am J Physiol 255:R344–R349, 1988

Keller-Wood ME, Shinsako J, Dallman MF: Inhibition of the adrenocorticotropin and corticosteroid responses to hypoglycemia after prior stress. Endocrinology 113:491–496, 1983

Knizley H: The hippocampus and septal area as primary target sites for corticosterone. J Neurochem 19:2737–2745, 1972

Kohno A, Seeman P, Cinader B: Age-related changes in beta-adrenoceptors in aging inbred mice. J Gerontol 41:439–444, 1986

Krauter EE, Wallace JE, Campbell BA: Sensory-motor function in the aging rat. Behav Neural Biol 31:367–392, 1981

Landfield PW: Hippocampal neurobiological mechanisms of age-related memory dysfunction. Neurobiol Aging 9:571–579, 1988

Landfield P, Waymire J, Lynch G: Hippocampal aging and adrenocorticoids: a quantitative correlation. Science 202:1098–1101, 1978

Levine S, Mullins RF: Hormonal influences on brain organization in infant rats. Science 152:1585–1592, 1966

Liddle GW: The adrenals, in Textbook of Endocrinology, 6th Edition. Edited by Williams RH. Philadelphia, PA, WB Saunders, 1981, pp 267–270

Liljequist S: Changes in the sensitivity of dopamine receptors in the nucleus accumbens and in the striatum. Acta Pharmacologica Toxicologica (Copenh) 43:19–28, 1978

Maggi A, Schmidt B, Ghetti B, et al: Effect of aging on neurotransmitter receptor binding in rat and human brain. Life Sci 24:367–377, 1979

Malamed S, Carsia RV: Aging of the rat adrenocortical cell: response to ACTH and cyclic AMP in vitro. J Gerontol 38:130–136, 1983

Marawaha J, Hoffer B, Pittman R, et al: Age-related electrophysiologic changes in rat cerebellum. Brain Res 201:85–97, 1980

Marshall JF: Sensorimotor disturbances in the aging rodent. J Gerontol 37:548–554, 1982

Marshall JF, Berrios N: Movement disorders of aged rats: reversal by dopamine receptor stimulation. Science 206:477–479, 1979

McCarty R: Aged rats: diminished sympathetic-adrenal medullary responses to acute stress. Behav Neural Biol 33:204–212, 1981

McCarty R: Effects of 2-Deoxyglucose on plasma catecholamines in adult and aged rats. Neurobiol Aging 5:285–289, 1984

McDonald RB, Horwitz BA, Stern JS: Cold-induced thermogenesis in younger and older Fischer 344 rats following exercise training. Am J Physiol 254:R908–R916, 1988

Middaugh LD, Ingram DK, Reynolds MA: Methadone effects on locomotor activity of young and aged mice. Neurobiol Aging 4:157–161, 1983

Miller M: Increased Vasopressin secretion: an early manifestation of aging in the rat. J Gerontol 42:3–7, 1987

Miquel J, Blasco M: A simple technique for evaluation of vitality loss in aging mice, by testing their muscle coordination and vigor. Exp Gerontol 13:389–396, 1976

Missale C, Govoni L, Croce A, et al: Changes of beta-endorphin and met-enkephalin content in the hypothalamus-pituitary-axis induced by aging. J Neurochem 40:20–25, 1983

Morley JE, Levine AS: Dynorphin (1-13) induces spontaneous feeding in rats. Life Sci 29:1901–1903, 1981

Munck A, Guyre P, Holbrook N: Physiological functions of glucocorticoids during stress and their relation to pharmacological actions. Endocr Rev 5:25–49, 1984

Naumenko EV, Maslova LN, Markel AL: Correction of arterial blood pressure in adult rats with inherited stress-induced hypertension by enhancement of catecholamine metabolism in early postnatal period. Endocrinol Exp 24:241–248, 1990

Nelson JF, Holinka CF, Lattham KR, et al: Corticosterone binding in cytosols from brain regions of mature and senescent male C57Bl/6J mice. Brain Res 115:345–351, 1976

Odio M, Brodish A: Effects of age on metabolic responses to acute and chronic stress. Am J Physiol 254:E617–E624, 1988

Odio M, Brodish A: Age-dependent effects of chronic stress on ACTH and corticosterone responses to an acute novel stress. Neuroendocrinology 49:496–501, 1989a

Odio M, Brodish A: Age-related adaptation of pituitary-adrenocortical responses to stress. Neuroendocrinology 49:382–388, 1989b

Okwusidi JI, Wong HY, Cheng KS, et al: Effects of diazepam, psychosocial stress and dietary cholesterol on pituitary-adrenocortical hormone levels and experimental atherosclerosis. Artery 18:71–86, 1991

Oxenkrug G, McIntyre M, Stanley M, et al: Dexamethasone suppression test: experimental model in rats, and effect of age. Biol Psychol 19:413–417, 1984

Pare WP: The effect of chronic environmental stress on premature aging in the rat. J Gerontol 20:78–84, 1965

Pfeifer WD, Davis LC: Modification of the adrenal stress response by age and prior experience. Exp Aging Res 2:27–36, 1975

Pittman RN, Minneman KP, Molinoff PB: Alterations in beta 1 and beta 2 adrenergic receptor density in the cerebellum of aging rats. J Neurochem 35:273–275, 1980

Ponzio F, Brunelo N, Algeri S: Catecholamine synthesis in brain of aging rat. J Neurochem 30:1617–1620, 1978

Popplewell PY, Tsubokawa M, Ramachandran J, et al: Differential effects of aging on adrenocorticotropin receptors, adenosine 3'5'-monophosphate response, and corticosterone secretion in adrenocortical cells from Sprague-Dawley rats. Endocrinology 119:2206–2213, 1986

Ratner A, Yelvington DB, Rosenthal MJ: Prolactin and corticosterone response to repeated foot shock stress in male rats. Psychoneuroendocrinology 114:393–396, 1989

Rattner BA, Michael SD, Altland PD: Age-related responses to mild restraint in the rat. J Appl Physiol 55:1408–1412, 1983

Reaven E, Kostrna M, Ramachandran J, et al: Structure and function changes in rat adrenal glands during aging. Am J Physiol 255:E903–E911, 1988

Rhees RW, Wilson CT, Heninger RW: Influence of streptozotocin diabetes and insulin therapy on plasma corticosterone levels in male rats. Horm Metab Res 15:353–354, 1983

Riegle GD: Chronic stress effects of adrenocortical responsiveness in young and aged rats. Neuroendocrinology 11:1–10, 1973

Riegle GD, Hess GD: Chronic and acute dexamethasone suppression of stress activation of the adrenal cortex in young and aged rats. Neuroendocrinology 9:175–187, 1972

Riegel G, Meites J: Effects of aging on LH and prolactin after LHRH, L-DOPA, methyl-DOPA and stress in male rats. Proc Soc Exp Biol Med 151:507–511, 1976

Ritter B: Effects of chronic restraints on open field activity of aging C57Bl/6J mice. Exp Aging Res 4:87–95, 1978

Rivier C, Brownstein M, Spiess J, et al: In vivo corticotropin releasing factor-induced secretion of adrenocorticotropin, β-endorphin and corticosterone. Endocrinology 110:272–278, 1982

Robinson DS: Changes in monoamine oxidase with aging. Federation Proceedings 34:103–107, 1975

Rosenthal MJ, Morley JE: Corticotropin releasing factor (CRF) and age-related differences in behavior of mice. Neurobiol Aging 10:167–171, 1989

Rosenthal MJ, Morley JE, Flood JF, et al: Relationship between behavioral and motor responses of mature and old mice and cerebellar beta-adrenergic receptor density. Mech Aging Dev 45:231–237, 1988

Rosenthal MJ, Varela M, Garcia A, et al: Age-related changes in the motor response to environmental novelty in the rat. Exp Gerontol 24:149–157, 1989

Roth GS: Brain dopaminergic and opiate receptors and responsiveness during aging, in Aging Brain and Ergot Alkaloids. Edited by Agnoli A. New York, Raven, 1983, pp 53–60

Sapolsky RM, Krey LC, McEwen B: The adreno-cortical stress-response in the aged male rat: impairment of recovery from stress. Exp Gerontol 18:55–64, 1983a

Sapolsky R, Krey L, McEwen B: Corticosterone receptors decline in a site-specific manner in the aged brain. Brain Res 289:235–240, 1983b

Sapolsky RM, Krey LC, McEwen BS: The neuroendocrinology of stress and aging: the glucocorticoid cascade hypothesis. Endocr Rev 7:284–301, 1986b

Scaccianoce S, Di Sciullo A, Anglelucci L: Age-related changes in hypothalamo-pituitary-adrenocortical axis activity in the rat. Neuroendocrinology 52:150–155, 1990

Schulze G, Janicke B: Effects of chronic hypaxis on behavioral and pathophysiological parameters. Neurobiol Aging 7:199–203, 1986

Sonntag WE, Steger RW, Forman LJ, et al: Decreased pulsatile release of growth hormone in old male rats. Endocrinology 107:1875–1879, 1980

Sonntag WE, Forman LJ, Miki N, et al: L-DOPA restores the amplitude of growth hormone pulses in old male rats to that observed in young male rats. Neuroendocrinology 34:163–168, 1982

Sonntag WE, Hylka W, Meites J: Impaired ability of old male rats to secrete GH in vivo but not in vitro in response to GRF 1-44. Endocrinology 113:2305–2307, 1983

Sonntag WE, Goliszek AG, Brodis A, et al: Diminished diurnal secretion of adrenocorticotropin (ACTH) but not corticosterone, in old male rats: possible relation to increased adrenal sensitivity to ACTH in vivo. 120:2308–2315, 1987

Sprott RL, Eleftheriou BE: Open field behavior in aging inbred mice. Gerontologia 20:155–160, 1974

Swenson RM, Vogel WH: Plasma catecholamines and corticosterone as well as brain catecholamine changes during coping in rats exposed to stressful footshock. Pharmacol Biochem Behav 18:689–693, 1983

Swerdlow NR, Vaccarino FJ, Androic M, et al: The neural substrates for the motor activating properties of psychostimulants. Pharmacol Biochem Behav 25:223–248, 1986

Tang F, Phillips JG: Some age-related changes in pituitary-adrenal function in the male laboratory rat. J Gerontol 33:377–382, 1978

Taylor J, Weyers P, Harris N, et al: The plasma catecholamine stress response is characteristic for a given animal over one-year period. Physiol Behav 46:853–856, 1989

Thurmond JB, Heishman SJ: Effect of catecholamine precursors on stress-induced changes in motor activity, exploration, and brain monoamines in young and aged mice. Behav Neurosci 98:506–517, 1984

Timiras PS: Biological perspectives on aging. American Scientist 35:364–370, 1978

Tornello S, Fridman O, Weisenberg L, et al: Differences in corticosterone binding by regions of the central nervous system in normal and diabetic rats. J Steroid Biochem 14:77–81, 1981

Verkhratski I, Didenko SO, Kharazi LI: Regulation of corticoliberin and corticotropin incretion in old age. Fiziol Zh 36:76–81, 1990

Walker JG, Walker JP: Neurohumoral regulation of adenylate cyclase activity in rat striatum. Brain Res 54:391–396, 1973

Wallace JE, Krauter EE, Campbell BA: Motor and reflexive behavior in the aging rat. J Gerontol 35:364–370, 1980

Watanabe H: Differential decrease in the rate of dopamine synthesis in several dopaminergic neurons in aged brain. Exp Gerontol 22:17–25, 1987

Welsh KA, Gold PE: Age-related changes in brain catecholamine responses to a single footshock. Neurobiol Aging 5:55–59, 1984

Wexler BC: Corticotropin stimulation of hypertensive rats with and without arteriosclerosis. Arch Pathol Lab Med 102:587–591, 1978

Wilson MM, Keith LD, Levitt GR, et al: Altered regulation of the pituitary-adrenal system of female rats during aging. Gerontologist 21:238–241, 1981

Yelvington DB, Rosenthal MJ, Ratner A: Effect of illness on hormonal response to footshock stress. Proc Soc Exp Biol Med 184:239–242, 1987

Yu BP, Bertrand HA, Masoro EJ: Nutrition-aging influence on catecholamine promoted lipolysis. Metab Clin Exp 29:438–444, 1980

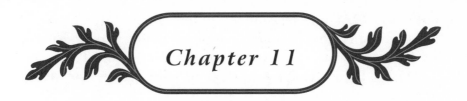

Chapter 11

Conclusions and Directions for Further Research

Paul E. Ruskin, M.D., and
John A. Talbott, M.D.

Although much has been learned about post-traumatic stress disorder (PTSD) and aging, much remains to be discovered. In the following brief summary, we delineate areas of current knowledge and provide directions for future research.

Late-Life Effects of Earlier Trauma

There is now a growing body of evidence from case reports and clinical research that PTSD can continue or can reoccur as long as 50 years after the initial trauma. This evidence comes predominantly from studies of World War II combat veterans (Christenson et al. 1981; Hamilton 1982; Van Dyke et al. 1985), prisoners of war (Goldstein et al. 1987; Kluznik et al. 1986; Zeiss and Dickman 1989), Holocaust survivors (Kuch and Cox 1992), and resistance fighters. In a study of Jewish Holocaust survivors who applied for German war reparations, for instance, Kuch and Cox found a 46% rate of current PTSD by DSM-III-R (American Psychiatric Association 1987) criteria.

Aarts et al. (Chapter 4) found a rate of 56% current PTSD among Dutch resistance fighters who were receiving a disability pension, and 25% among those not receiving a pension. Clearly, severe emotional trauma can have long-lasting effects into old age. Kuch and Cox found that the rate of PTSD was three times as great among survivors of Auschwitz (65%) compared with survivors who had not been in concentration camps (22%), suggesting that the severity of the original trauma is positively correlated with the rate of late-life PTSD.

PTSD can follow a number of different patterns over time. There are numerous clinical reports that describe the recurrence or emergence of PTSD in later life (Christenson et al. 1981; Hamilton 1982; Van Dyke et al. 1985). These reports suggest that late-life stressors such as the death of a spouse, retirement, or physical illness can precipitate the recurrence or onset of PTSD symptoms. Two explanations for these phenomena have been postulated. First, it has been suggested that late-life events such as physical illness or the death of loved ones is symbolically representative of the traumatic period when the threat of death or injury was present. These late-life events could therefore trigger an emotional reliving of the original trauma. Second, it has been postulated that trauma victims repress the trauma by working hard, raising children, and so on. With retirement and the leaving of children, the victim has more time to think about the trauma. Unfortunately, there are no well-controlled studies that demonstrate 1) that symptoms of PTSD occur more commonly in elderly persons who experience late-life stressors than in elderly persons who do not experience such stress or 2) that symptoms increase as former trauma victims enter old age. Longitudinal studies, such as those conducted by Clipp and Elder (Chapter 3) are needed to answer these questions definitively.

Investigators have examined the prevalence of symptoms such as anxiety and depression among elderly individuals who experienced severe trauma earlier in life. Randomly designed studies of nonclinical samples of Holocaust survivors indicate that the overall level of symptomatology is greater than among a control group (Kahana et al. 1989). Severity of trauma has been correlated with extent of symptoms in almost all studies. Clipp and Elder's (Chapter 3) longitudinal study presents evidence that, overall, symptoms decrease over time. Survivors of severe trauma are a heterogeneous group. Whereas some manifest long-term psychological symptoms as a result of the trauma, others demonstrate no trauma-related symptoms. Sigal and Weinfeld (1989) found that 64% of male and 35% of female Holocaust survivors "did not give evidence of psychiatric impairment" according to the cutoff criterion they used for their rating scale (p. 163).

A few studies have looked at the rate of psychosomatic illness among Holocaust survivors. Stermer et al. (1991), for instance, found a significantly higher rate of chronic functional gastrointestinal symptoms among Holocaust survivors than among control subjects. Kahana et al. (1989) reported that Holocaust survivors were more likely than control subjects to report psychogenic symptoms.

Quality of social functioning has also been studied. Robinson et al. (1990) interviewed 86 Holocaust survivors and concluded that "they are successful at work and in society. They managed to raise warm families" (p. 311). Sigal and Weinfeld (1989) found that Holocaust survivors living in Montreal "seemed reasonably well adjusted both sociopolitically and economically" (p. 164). Kahana et al. (1989) found that Holocaust survivors had higher income, superior job histories, greater residential stability, and lower divorce rates than a control group. Survivors were also noted to be more active in their communities and to "portray significantly higher levels of altruism" (p. 205). Harel et al. (1988) found that Holocaust survivors had significantly higher levels of coping than a control group, as well as higher levels of communication with their children. Thus, it would appear that despite an increase in psychiatric symptoms, survivors are able to maintain a level of social functioning that is equal or even better than nonsurvivors.

Kaminer and Lavie (1991) compared sleep of well-adjusted Holocaust survivors, less-adjusted survivors, and a control group. The less-adjusted survivors had more prolonged sleep latency, lower sleep efficiency, and more dream recall than the other two groups. Aarts et al. (Chapter 4) found that among former resistance fighters, subjects with current PTSD had a decrease of total sleep time, sleep efficiency, rapid-eye-movement-sleep latency, and deep sleep (stages III-IV). Thus, it appears that there can be a disruption of sleep in later years as a result of trauma suffered years before.

Clipp and Elder (Chapter 3) report a strong relationship between premorbid psychological functioning and the development of war-related symptoms. Subjects with poor psychological adjustment during adolescence tended to have greater emotional reactions to combat. Further study of premorbid functioning as a predictor of later emotional dysfunction is important but very difficult to achieve due to the methodological problems involved in obtaining premorbid data.

Clipp and Elder (Chapter 3) also report interesting data on the relationship between age at time of trauma to subsequent psychological and social functioning. Subjects who were younger (late teens and early 20s) during combat had more symptoms of emotional distress at the time of the war and in subsequent years than those who were older (late 20s and early 30s). On the other hand, the older subjects had marked socioeconomic disadvantages lasting into late life as a result of the disruption of their careers and marriages by the war. Studies of child survivors of the Holocaust indicate that they have higher rates of psychological symptoms than individuals who had reached adulthood by the time of the war (Dasberg 1987). On the other hand, child survivors manifest a high level of professional and social functioning. Thus it would seem that although trauma at a younger age might lead to greater psychological symptoms over time, it might not result in greater functional impairment.

A few studies have looked at the emotional reaction of survivors to current traumatic situations. Eaton et al. (1982), for instance, found that Holocaust survivors were more sensitive to the rising anti-Semitism in Montreal during the 1970s than a control group. Solomon and Prager (1992) found that during the Gulf War, "Holocaust survivors perceived higher levels of danger and reported more symptoms of acute distress than comparison subjects. In addition, they displayed higher levels of both state and trait anxiety" (p. 1707). Baider et al. (1992) compared Holocaust survivors with cancer to a control group of cancer patients who were not Holocaust survivors. The survivors "were unable to mobilize partial denial and their psychological distress was much higher. Their functioning, however, did not significantly differ from that of the comparison group" (p. 11). Thus, it would seem that survivors respond with increased symptomatology to psychological stress in later life.

The work of Clipp and Elder (Chapter 3) indicates that veterans who have received emotional support from wives and former comrades had lower rates of psychological distress over time that those who did not have a strong social support system. Fenig and Levav (1991) found that among Holocaust survivors, demoralization was inversely related to the amount of current social support. Harel et al. (1988) also found that high levels of social support were inversely proportional to psychological symptoms. In fact, this study indicated that good physical health, adequate economic resources, and being married led to better psychological health among survivors in later years. In summary, it would seem that high levels of social support mitigate the late-life effects of early trauma.

A few studies have examined the benefits—as well as the obvious liabilities—of having suffered from severe emotional trauma. Clipp and Elder (Chapter 3), for instance, found that "developmental change toward greater self-direction, confidence, and assertiveness characterized the early entrants compared with late entrants and nonveterans" (p. 42).

There have been no well-controlled studies of the best methods of treatment for elderly patients who manifest PTSD as a result of trauma suffered years before. Should patients attempt to recapture repressed unpleasant memories after so many years, or is it better for them to try to forget intrusive thoughts? The best type of psychotherapeutic treatment—group, individual, or behavioral—has not been determined, nor has the role of psychotropic medication.

Effects of Late-Life Trauma

Fields (Chapter 5) provides a comprehensive summary of research concerning the psychological effects of late-life trauma. He concludes that compared with younger individuals, the elderly suffer the same, or even lower, rates of PTSD and other psychological symptoms when exposed to severe trauma. He adds that premorbid level of psychological functioning and the severity of the trauma are much more important predictors of symptomatology than age. Finally, he suggests that "as a group, the elderly [trauma victims] ask less, complain less, and receive less in resources than younger-age ranges of the population" (p. 96).

Green et al. (Chapter 6) found that the elderly manifested less psychological distress to the Buffalo Creek flood than younger age groups. In fact, people who were middle age were the most symptomatic. These age differences were still apparent 14 years after the flood, although overall levels of distress had decreased in all age groups. Green et al. found that the elderly utilized different methods of coping with the disaster than younger individuals. "The subjects in our two older age groups reported much higher rates than other age groups of turning to religion to cope with their distress about the disaster. Similarly, they were more likely to spend their leisure time attending church than the younger subjects" (p. 134).

Goldstein (Chapter 7) proposes that elder abuse can be a precipitant for PTSD in the elderly. She suggests an expansion of the diagnostic criteria for PTSD to include symptoms that are commonly observed in the abused elderly.

> In the elderly maltreated person, the "intensive fear, help-lessness, or horror" ([American Psychiatric Association 1994] p. 428) can manifest itself also by "disorganized or agitated behavior" (p. 428). . . . Especially in an older de-mented individual, the content of the reexperienced trauma may be expressed in the form of a delusion with-out ability to recall the actual facts. Manifestations of the trauma of neglect include malnutrition, dehydration, de-lirium, signs of inadequate or excessive hearing, and the absence of prosthetic aids where needed. . . . Manifesta-tions of abuse of the use of medications, prescribed or over the counter, could include a state of delirium, memory impairment, agitation, lethargy, and self-neglect. . . . Avoiding "activities, places, or people that arouse recollec-tions of the trauma" (American Psychiatric Association 1994, p. 428) may manifest itself by avoiding the infor-mal or formal provider of care. The feeling of life being over—"sense of a foreshortened future" (p. 428)—may be perceived as "normal" in an 80-year-old person by those unaware of the abuse or course of the aging process (pp. 148).

Models of Stress and the Elderly

Life Events

An extensive literature documents the relationship between negative life events and depression in the elderly (George 1989). Bereavement, for instance, is highly related to depres-sion, as is poor physical health.

Guarnaccia and Zautra (Chapter 8) found that there is a greater degree of psychological disturbance following the onset of physical disability than as a result of conjugal bereavement. The disabled group manifested significantly more depression and anxiety than the control group, whereas the bereaved group manifested only more depression than control subjects. Psychological distress persisted more over time in the disabled than in the bereaved group. Furthermore, the disabled had more undesirable small events in their daily lives. This might be a mechanism to explain the ongoing symptomatology of this group. Finally, subjects who were actively engaged in coping with bereavement or disability experienced less psychological distress than other subjects.

Guarnaccia and Zautra (Chapter 8) suggest that the conceptual and methodological framework of general stress research be applied more to PTSD research. "It may be beneficial to study the negative small life events of those with PTSD" (p. 173).

Physiological Response to Stress

In contrast to the similarity between the old and young in psychological response to negative life events, there are major physiological differences in response to mild stress. McNeilly and Anderson (Chapter 9) note that compared with younger individuals, the elderly respond with less increase in heart rate, greater blood pressure reactivity, decreased skin conductive levels, greater increase in catecholamines with a longer return to baseline levels, and decreased beta-adrenergic activity.

Rosenthal (Chapter 10) notes numerous differences between younger and older animals in response to stress. Certain stress-related behaviors are decreased in older animals, and others are increased. Differences were also observed in central catecholamine, and possibly also in peripheral catecholamine, response. Rosenthal concludes that "although corticosterone responses to stress are well sustained in older rodents, central control of the adrenal-pituitary axis is impaired in older animals" (p. 242). He reports changes in luteinizing hormone and growth hormone, but not prolactin, in old compared to young rodents exposed to stress. Rosenthal concludes that,

> By and large, older animals are able to mount successful responses during stressful arousal despite the loss of cer-

tain components of that response. However, when faced with maximal stimulation, older animals manage poorly. Maximal responses are diminished, and mortality is increased. This response pattern occurs with a number of behavioral and hormonal indicators. (p. 254)

Conclusion

Research to date provides conflicting evidence concerning the vulnerability of older people to severe stress. On the one hand, it seems that elderly people are no more—and possibly less—vulnerable to the psychological effects of severe trauma than are younger individuals. Furthermore, the elderly are no more sensitive to negative life events.

On the other hand, there is anecdotal evidence that late-life stressors can cause a recurrence of symptoms related to early trauma. Further research is necessary to validate this clinical impression.

Finally, studies of human response to mild stress, and animal response to greater stress, suggest that the elderly respond differently physiologically to stress than the young. The exact relationship between these physiological differences and the development of PTSD is as yet unknown. Further research is necessary to make this link.

References

American Psychiatric Association: Diagnostic and Statistical Manual of Mental Disorders, 3rd Edition, Revised. Washington, DC, American Psychiatric Association, 1987

American Psychiatric Association: Diagnostic and Statistical Manual of Mental Disorders, 4th Edition. Washington, DC, American Psychiatric Association, 1994

Baider L, Peretz T, De-Nour AK: Effect of the Holocaust on coping with cancer. Soc Sci Med 34:11–15, 1992

Christenson RM, Walker JI, Ross DR, et al: Reactivation of traumatic conflicts. Am J Psychiatry 138:984–985, 1981

Dasberg H: Psychological distress of Holocaust survivors and offspring in Israel, forty years later: a review. Isr J Psychiatry Relat Sci 24:243–256, 1987

Eaton WW, Sigal JJ, Weinfeld M: Impairment in Holocaust survivors after 33 years: data from an unbiased community sample. Am J Psychiatry 139:773–777, 1982

Fenig S, Levav I: Demoralization and social supports among Holocaust survivors. J Nerv Ment Dis 179:167–172, 1991

George LK: Stress, social support, and depression over the life-course, in Aging, Stress, and Health. Edited by Markides KS, Cooper CL. New York, Wiley, 1989, pp 241–261

Goldstein G, van Kammer W, Shelly C, et al: Survivors of imprisonment in the Pacific theater during World War II. Am J Psychiatry 144:1210–1213, 1987

Hamilton JW: Unusual long-term sequelae of a traumatic war experience. Bull Menninger Clin 46:539–541, 1982

Harel Z, Kahana B, Kahana E: Psychological well-being among Holocaust survivors and immigrants in Israel. Journal of Traumatic Stress 1:413–429, 1988

Kahana B, Harel Z, Kahana E: Clinical and gerontological issues facing survivors of the Nazi Holocaust, in Healing Their Wounds: Psychotherapy With the Holocaust Survivors and Their Families. Edited by Marcu P, Rosenberg A. New York, Praeger, 1989, pp 197–211

Kaminer H, Lavie P: Sleep and dreaming in Holocaust survivors: dramatic decrease in dream recall in well-adjusted survivors. J Nerv Ment Dis 179:664–669, 1991

Kluznik JC, Speed N, VanValkenburg C, et al: Forty-year follow-up of United States prisoners of war. Am J Psychiatry 143:1443–1446, 1986

Kuch K, Cox BJ: Symptoms of PTSD in 124 survivors of the Holocaust. Am J Psychiatry 149:337–340, 1992

Robinson S, Rapaport J, Durst R, et al: The late effects of Nazi persecution among elderly Holocaust survivors. Acta Psychiatr Scand 82:311–315, 1990

Sigal JJ, Weinfeld M. Trauma and Rebirth: Intergenerational Effects of the Holocaust. New York, Praeger, 1989

Solomon Z, Prager E: Elderly Israeli Holocaust survivors during the Persian Gulf War: a study of psychological distress. Am J Psychiatry 149:1707–1710, 1992

Stermer E, Bar H, Levy N: Chronic functional gastrointestinal symptoms in Holocaust survivors. Am J Gastroenterol 86:417–422, 1991

Van Dyke C, Zilberg NJ, McKinnon JA: Posttraumatic stress disorder: a thirty-year delay in a World War II veteran. Am J Psychiatry 142:1070–1073, 1985

Zeiss RA, Dickman HR: PTSD 40 years later: incidence and person-situation correlates in former POWs. J Clin Psychol 45:80–87, 1989

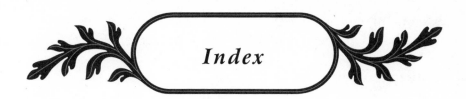

Index